New Horizons for Schistosomiasis Research

Edited by Tonay Inceboz

Published in London, United Kingdom

New Horizons for Schistosomiasis Research
http://dx.doi.org/10.5772/intechopen.95134
Edited by Tonay Inceboz

Contributors
Andressa Barban do Patrocínio, Benjamin Amoani, Gideon Kwesi Nakotey, Samuel Asamoah Sakyi, Karen Pomeyie, Christian Sewor, Genanew Birhanu, Célestin Kyambikwa Bisangamo, Tonay Inceboz

First published in London, United Kingdom, 2022 by IntechOpen
IntechOpen is the global imprint of INTECHOPEN LIMITED, registered in England and Wales, registration number: 11086078, 5 Princes Gate Court, London, SW7 2QJ, United Kingdom

British Library Cataloguing-in-Publication Data
A catalogue record for this book is available from the British Library

Additional hard and PDF copies can be obtained from orders@intechopen.com

New Horizons for Schistosomiasis Research
Edited by Tonay Inceboz
p. cm.

This title is part of the Infectious Diseases Book Series, Volume 14
Topic: Parasitic Infectious Diseases
Series Editor: Alfonso J. Rodriguez-Morales
Topic Editor: Amidou Samie

Print ISBN 978-1-80355-855-4
Online ISBN 978-1-80355-856-1
eBook (PDF) ISBN 978-1-80355-857-8
ISSN 2631-6188

IntechOpen Book Series

Infectious Diseases

Volume 14

Aims and Scope of the Series

This series will provide a comprehensive overview of recent research trends in various Infectious Diseases (as per the most recent Baltimore classification). Topics will include general overviews of infections, immunopathology, diagnosis, treatment, epidemiology, etiology, and current clinical recommendations for managing infectious diseases. Ongoing issues, recent advances, and future diagnostic approaches and therapeutic strategies will also be discussed. This book series will focus on various aspects and properties of infectious diseases whose deep understanding is essential for safeguarding the human race from losing resources and economies due to pathogens.

Meet the Series Editor

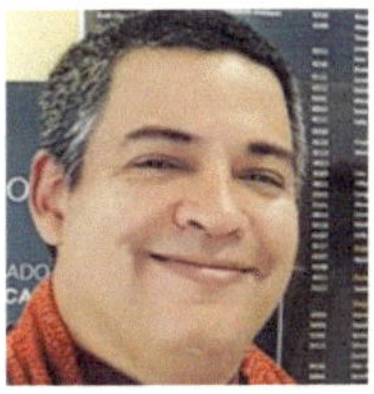

Dr. Rodriguez-Morales is an expert in tropical and emerging diseases, particularly zoonotic and vector-borne diseases (especially arboviral diseases). He is the president of the Travel Medicine Committee of the Pan-American Infectious Diseases Association (API), as well as the president of the Colombian Association of Infectious Diseases (ACIN). He is a member of the Committee on Tropical Medicine, Zoonoses, and Travel Medicine of ACIN. He is a vice-president of the Latin American Society for Travel Medicine (SLAMVI) and a Member of the Council of the International Society for Infectious Diseases (ISID). Since 2014, he has been recognized as a Senior Researcher, at the Ministry of Science of Colombia. He is a professor at the Faculty of Medicine of the Fundacion Universitaria Autonoma de las Americas, in Pereira, Risaralda, Colombia. He is an External Professor, Master in Research on Tropical Medicine and International Health, Universitat de Barcelona, Spain. He is also a professor at the Master in Clinical Epidemiology and Biostatistics, Universidad Científica del Sur, Lima, Peru. In 2021 he has been awarded the "Raul Isturiz Award" Medal of the API. Also, in 2021, he was awarded with the "Jose Felix Patiño" Asclepius Staff Medal of the Colombian Medical College, due to his scientific contributions to COVID-19 during the pandemic. He is currently the Editor in Chief of the journal Travel Medicine and Infectious Diseases. His Scopus H index is 47 (Google Scholar H index, 68).

Meet the Volume Editor

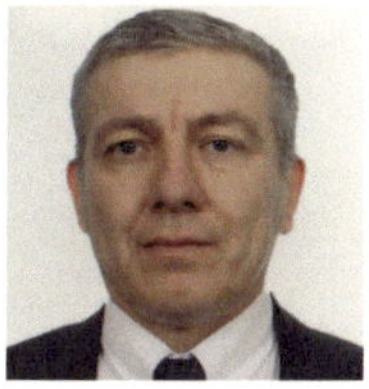

Tonay Inceboz is a senior lecturer in Medical Parasitology. He had his MD degree at Ege University Medical Faculty, Turkiye in 1988. He had his Ph.D. degree in Parasitology at the same university in 1998. He is currently a professor at the Department of Medical Parasitology, Medical Faculty, Dokuz Eylul University, Turkiye. His main research interests are *Entamoeba histolytica*, *Blastocystis hominis*, *Echinococcus granulosus*, *E. multilocularis, Trichomonas vaginalis*, and ticks. Prof. Inceboz has given many lectures and presentations at different academic meetings. He has more than sixty journal articles and nineteen book chapters to his credit. He is also an editor of one book.

Contents

Preface

Schistosomiasis (bilharziasis) is a parasitic disease caused by *Schistosoma* spp. that belongs to trematode worms. These worms are known as blood parasites. This disease is considered both a neglected tropical disease and a water-borne disease. The cardinal species are *Schistosoma haematobium* (1852), *S. japonicum* (1904), *S. mansoni* (1907), *S. intercalatum* (1934), *S. mekongi* (1978), *S. guineensis*, and *S. intercalatum*, though there are more than twenty different species overall. The parasite in the definitive host may affect many organs and systems, such as the liver, lungs, urogenital system, gastrointestinal tract, and so on. The disease may become chronic and last 3–8 years, and in some cases even up to 20–30 years.

According to the World Health Organization (WHO), schistosomiasis affects 250 million people, threatens 800 million people, and causes 1.9 million deaths yearly in endemic tropical and subtropical areas. Endemic areas include the Middle East, South America, Caribbean, Southeast Asia, and particularly sub-Saharan Africa. The definitive host is primarily human; however, in endemic areas a variety of animals such as monkeys, cattle, horses, rodents, cats, and dogs are also considered reservoirs. Moreover, due to global warming, the spread of the disease may increase. This level of incidence and urgency of schistosomiasis points to the importance of finding a remedy for this disease. A remedy would be beneficial not only for humans but also for animals worldwide. In addition, effective treatment and prevention will mitigate further socioeconomic losses, another consequence of the disease.

This book presents up-to-date information about schistosomiasis, including diagnosis, treatment, epidemiology, control, new molecular methods, and vaccine studies. We wish to thank the chapter authors for their excellent contributions.

Tonay Inceboz
The Department of Medical Parasitology,
Dokuz Eylul University of Medical Faculty,
İzmir, Türkiye

Chapter 1

Introductory Chapter: Changing Our Perspectives on Schistosomiasis

Tonay Inceboz

1. Introduction

Humanity in the 21st-century has made many scientific and cultural advancements. This development in technology improves people's living conditions [1]. However, the growth of technology also causes physical deterioration of nature via many chemical, nuclear, and solid wastes during the use of food and energy sources or pollution of water [2, 3]. The ecological balance of nature is being destroyed albeit unintentionally. This causes logarithmic growth and mutation of all kinds of microorganisms in the environment, resulting in the emergence of different species [4, 5].

Schistosomiasis is a term that denotes a disease caused by parasites belonging to genus *Schistosoma*. It is a major disease affecting approximately 250 million people in 78 countries and many regions in the world, mainly Asia, Africa, and America [6, 7]. There are more than 20 species of *Schistosoma* (*Schistosoma haematobium (S. haematobium)* (1852), *S. japonicum* (1904), *S. mansoni* (1907), *S. intercalatum* (1934), *S. mekongi* (1978), *S. guineensis* and *S. intercalatum* et al.) in the tropical and subtropical regions of the world.

Schistosoma spp. involve humans and certain animals (monkeys, rodents, cattle, etc.) as definitive hosts, and snails (*Biomphalaria*, *Bulinus*, *Oncomelania*, etc.) as intermediate hosts. Since cercaria forms of *Schistosoma* are disseminated via contaminated water, they spread far and wide. In fact, the history of schistosomiasis in humans goes back to ancient times [8]. *S. haematobium* eggs have been found in the kidneys of Egyptian mummies. However, the first description of schistosomiasis was made by the German pathologist Theodore Maximilian Bilharz (1825 to 1862) by autopsy examinations on infected patients in Egypt. He named the worm that recovered from the portal vein as "*Schistosoma hematobium*". Doctor Yoshinao Fujii (1818 to 1895) of Japan was described the symptoms of schistosomiasis. He noticed rush in the legs, fever, diarrhea and bloody stool among the villagers who worked in the trice fields of Katayama. In 1904, Fujiro Katsurada found the causative agent of Katayama fever and named the worm "*Schistosoma japonicum*". Three years later, in 1907, *S. mansoni* was discovered as the third type of *Schistosoma* by Luigi Westenra Sambon (1865 to 1931).

Although they have been known for years, the diagnosis, treatment, and prevention of schistosomiasis did not reach their full maturity. That is why it is still a major health problem in many countries. Even more, schistosomiasis has increased drastically and resulted in financial problems by causing chronic diseases [9]. In response to this, the World Health Organization (WHO) initiated a long-term program to fight against schistosomiasis with various methods, such as education and praziquantel therapy, by launching an extensive project [10].

2. Conclusions

It is important to note once again that *Schistosoma* spp. are often seen in socio-economically underdeveloped regions. When dealing with *Schistosoma* spp., the intermediate hosts (the snails), the definitive hosts (humans and certain animal species), and the source of infection (infective waters) should be considered [11, 12].

When we look deeper into Schistosomiasis we find that the disease can be in two phases: acute and chronic. *Schistosoma* may involve many organs in the body by dissemination via bloodstream. Symptoms may vary according to involved organs. In the acute phase; high fever, Katayama fever (specific for *Schistosoma japonicum and S. mansoni*), myalgia, fatigue, abdominal pain, diarrhea, haematuria may be present. However, in chronic phase of schistosomiasis, different symptoms, due to more specific organ infoldments, can be found such as hepatosplenomegaly, gastrointestinal bleeding, and abdominal pain due to ascites and periportal fibrosis, bladder carcinoma (specific for *Schistosoma hematobium*), etc. Long-term consequences can also lead to socio-economic burden, such as dependent life and long-term treatment costs [13].

The diagnosis of schistosomiasis is not always easy in humans. History taking is very important to "think about" the disease in differential diagnosis. Laboratory tests such as antigen (circulating cathodic antigen (CCA)) or antibody tests are the most commonly used tests in diagnosis. However, these are not "gold standard test" [14, 15]. The Kato-Katz technique (antigen) is a stool screening method (38% sensitivity) because it is the fastest and cheapest method [14, 16]. Serological techniques antigen tests (ELISA, IHA, and IFAT) are widely used for the diagnosis of schistosomiasis [17]. The diagnosis of *S. japonicum* is made by PCR (52% of the PCR positive samples were positive) [14] and PCR ELISA for *S. mansoni* (sensitivity was high (97.4%), and the specificity was more satisfactory (85.1%)) [18]. The commonly recommended treatment of schistosomiasis is praziquantel [19]. There have been many medications tested against schistosomiasis but still, there is not any good alternative in use to praziquantel.

Putting the treatment of schistosomiasis aside, we should focus on the prevention of the disease all over the world, and especially in endemic regions. We should consider that the disturbance of ecologic balance might cause new species of *Schistosoma*, newly infected water basins, and snail types [20]. It may be more difficult to cope with these new forms.

In this book, we all aimed to draw attention to "schistosomiasis" and how we can change our perspectives to "combat" and -hopefully- eradicate this important parasite disease. To overcome schistosomiasis globally, we should make endeavor to respect nature to avoid disturbing the ecological balance, to perform new scientific multidisciplinary studies, and to work as one, as in the "One Health" concept.

Author details

Tonay Inceboz
Department of Parasitology, Dokuz Eylul University, Medical Faculty, Turkiye

*Address all correspondence to: tonay.inceboz@gmail.com

References

[1] Zhou Y, Liu Y, Wu W. Strengthen China's flood control. Nature. 2016;**536**:396. DOI: 10.1038/536396e

[2] Knight M, Wu JY, Zhou YB, Chen Y, Liang S, Li LH, et al. Three gorges Dam: Impact of water level changes on the density of schistosome-transmitting snail Oncomelania hupensis in Dongting Lake area, China. PLoS Neglected Tropical Diseases. 2015;**9**:e0003882. DOI: 10.1371/journal.pntd.0003882

[3] Steinmann P, Keiser J, Bos R, Tanner M, Utzinger J. Schistosomiasis and water resources development: Systematic review, meta-analysis, and estimates of people at risk. The Lancet Infectious Diseases. 2006;**6**:411-425. DOI: 10.1016/S1473-3099(06)70521-7

[4] Chen W, Yang X, Huang X, Zhang Y, Cai S, Liu J, et al. Influence of flood in 1998 on schistosomiasis epidemic. Chinese Journal of Schistosomiasis Control. 2000;**12**:202-205. DOI: 10.16250/j.32.1374.2000.04.005 (In Chinese)

[5] Diaz JH. Rodent-borne infectious disease outbreaks after flooding disasters: Epidemiology, management, and prevention. Journal of Emergency Management. 2015;**13**:459-467. DOI: 10.5055/jem.2015.0255

[6] World Health Organization. Schistosomiasis (Bilharzia). Available online:https://www.who.int/health-topics/schistosomiasis#tab=tab_1. [Accessed: June 6, 2022]

[7] https://apps.who.int/neglected_diseases/ntddata/sch/sch.html. [Accessed: June 6, 2022]

[8] Ruffer MA. Note on the presence of "bilharzia haematobia" in Eqyptian mummies of the twentieth dynasty. British Medical Journal. 1910;**1**:16 https://www.ncbi.nlm.nih.gov/pmc/articles/PMC2330583/pdf/brmedj07759-0017b.pdf. [Accessed: July 13, 2022

[9] Silva-Moraes V, Shollenberger LM, Siqueira LMV, Castro-Borges W, Harn DA, Grenfell RFQE, et al. Diagnosis of Schistosoma Mansoni infections: What are the choices in Brazilian low-endemic areas? Memorias Do Instituto Oswaldo Cruz. 2019;**114**:2. DOI: 10.1590/0074-02760180478

[10] Schistosomiasis: progress report 2001-2011 and strategic plan 2012-2020. Assembly WHO. Elimination of Schistosomiasis. WHA65.21. 2012. file:///C:/Users/TM%C3%9C2/Downloads/9789241503174_eng.pdf. [Accessed: June 6, 2022]

[11] Rossati A. Global warming and its health impact. The International Journal of Occupational and Environmental Medicine. 2017;**8**:7-20. DOI: 10.15171/ijoem.2017.963

[12] Cao C, Li S, Zhou X. Impact of schistosomiasis transmission by catastrophic flood damage and emergency response in China. Chinese Journal of Schistosomiasis Control. 2016;**28**:618-623. DOI: 10.16250/j.32.1374.2016215

[13] Giorgio S, Gallo-Francisco PH, Roque GAS, Flóro e Silva M. Granulomas in parasitic diseases: The good and the bad. Parasitology Research. 2020;**119**(10):3165-3180. DOI: 10.1007/s00436-020-06841-x

[14] Lier T, Simonsen GS, Wang T, Lu D, Haukland HH, Vennervald BJ, et al. Real time polymerase chain reaction for

detection of low intensity *Schistosoms japonicum* infections in China. The American Journal of Tropical Medicine and Hygiene. 2009;**81**:428-432. DOI: 10.4269/ajtmh.2009.81.428

[15] Van Dam GJ, Wichers JH, Ferrera TM, Ghati D, Van Amerongen A, Deelder AM. Diagnosis of schistosomiasis by reagent strip test for detection of circulating cathodic antigen. Journal of Clinical Microbiology. 2004;**42**:5458-5461. DOI: 10.1128/JCM.42.12.5458-5461.2004

[16] Katz N, Chaves A, Pellegrino J. A simple device for quantitative stool thick smear technique in Schistosoma mansoni. Revista do Instituto de Medicina Tropical de Sao Paulo. 1972;**14**:397-400

[17] Gryseels B, Polman K, Clerinx J, Kestens L. Human schistosomiasis. Lancet. 2006;**368**:1106-1118. DOI: 10.1016/S0140-6736(06)69440-3

[18] Gomes LI, Marques LHS, Enk MJ, de Oliveira MC, Coelho PMZ, et al. Development and evaluation of a sensitive PCR-ELISA system for detection of *Schistosoma* infection in feces. PLoS Neglected Tropical Diseases. 2010;**4**(4):e664. DOI: 10.1371/journal.pntd.0000664

[19] Tchuenté LA, Shaw DJ, Polla L, Cioli D, Vercruysse J. Efficacy of praziquantel against *Schistosoma* haematobium infection in children. The American Journal of Tropical Medicine and Hygiene. 2004;**71**(6):778-782. DOI: 10.4269/ajtmh.2004.71.778

[20] Kamel B, Laidemitt MR, Lu L, Babbitt C, Weinbaum OL, Mkoji GM, et al. Detecting and identifying *Schistosoma* infections in snails andaquatic habitats: A systematic review. PLoS Neglected Tropical Diseases. 2021;**15**(3):e0009175. DOI: 10.1371/journal.pntd.0009175

Chapter 2

Epidemiology and Control of Schistosomiasis

Célestin Kyambikwa Bisangamo

Abstract

Human schistosomiasis is caused by the genus *Schistosoma*. Its prevalence and morbidity are highest among schoolchildren, adolescents, and young adults. It is prevalent in poor communities without access to safe drinking water and adequate sanitation. The agents of etiology of these diseases are *Schistosoma mansoni, Schistosoma haematobium, Schistosoma guineensis, Schistosoma intercalatum, Schistosoma japonicum, and Schistosoma mekongi*. Symptoms include anemia, stunting, fever, cough, abdominal pain, diarrhea, hepatosplenomegaly, genital lesions, and eosinophilia. Freshwater mollusks are suitable intermediate hosts, and the definitive hosts are the parasitized men. The transmission gap of disease is bridged when people come into contact with unwholesome water sources infested. People are infected through their usual agricultural, domestic, professional, or recreational activities, which expose them to contaminated water. Various animals, such as cattle, dogs, cats, rodents, pigs, horses, and goats, serve as reservoirs. Treatment of at-risk people on a wide scale, access to good water, improved sanitation, hygiene education, and snail control are all used to combat schistosomiasis. The WHO's schistosomiasis control strategy focuses on reducing disease by regularly administering praziquantel to affected populations on a large scale. It entails the regular treatment of all at-risk populations. Disease transmission should be halted in specific countries where transmission is low.

Keywords: schistosomiasis, epidemiology, prevention, control

1. Introduction

Human schistosomiasis (or bilharzia) is a chronic disease caused by parasitic worms. It is a parasitic neglected tropical disease and remains, after malaria, one of the main sources of morbidity and mortality in high prevalence countries, with major consequences on the health of the population and the economy [1].

According to the World Health Organization (WHO), 207 million people may have schistosomiasis in the world [2]. In 2018, it was estimated that at least 229 million people needed preventive treatment for schistosomiasis, while the number of people treated was 97.2 million [3].

Ninety percent of the disease burden is in sub-Saharan Africa, where the main species that cause schistosomiasis in humans are *Schistosoma mansoni* (intestinal schistosomiasis) and *S. haematobium* (urogenital schistosomiasis), which are transmitted through feces and urine, respectively [4, 5].

Victims are infected through their usual agricultural, domestic, professional, or recreational activities, which expose them to contaminated water. Lack of hygiene and certain play habits of school-age children, such as swimming or fishing in infested waters, make these children particularly vulnerable to infection [3].

Symptoms of schistosomiasis include anemia, stunting, fever, genital lesions, and irreversible organ damage [6–8].

The fight against schistosomiasis aims to reduce the number of patients by means of periodic large-scale treatment of populations with praziquantel; a more comprehensive approach, including access to drinking water, appropriate sanitation and the fight against gastropods, should also reduce the transmission of schistosomiasis [3].

The WHO recommends praziquantel-based preventive chemotherapy for schistosomiasis control; this treatment is given largely to school-aged children aged 5 to 15, who have the largest infection burden and may be reached efficiently through schools [9]. The prevention chemotherapeutic strategy is defined by the prevalence of schistosomiasis in the implementation unit (usually the district). A prevalence of schistosomiasis <10% entails the administration of preventive chemotherapy every 3 years; 10 to 49%, treatment every 2 years; and ≥ 50%, treatment annually [10]. The initial success in the prevention and control of schistosomiasis in some countries [11] had led to the WHO's more ambitious vision of "a world with zero cases of schistosomiasis infection" [12].

The WHO set goals to reduce schistosomiasis morbidity (referred to as disease control; defined as a heavy-intensity prevalence of infection of less than 5% aggregated across sentinel sites) by 2020 and eliminate schistosomiasis as a public health problem (referred to as elimination; defined as a prevalence of heavy-intensity infection of less than 1% in all sentinel sites) by 2025 in countries where human schistosomias By 2025, it is also hoped to have completely stopped the spread of schistosomiasis in some areas [12–14].

The WHO's strategic plan provides guidance on how programs can move from control of schistosomiasis to elimination and interruption of transmission [12].

Owing to epidemiologic and endemicity heterogeneities of schistosomiasis, one may predict that the timelines for transitioning between goals will not be uniform across all countries.

As a result, quantitative data from program monitoring must be analyzed to evaluate and improve these standards. According to recent theoretical modeling, the 2020 disease control goal outlined in the current treatment guideline is likely to be met in areas with low or moderate prevalence but will be missed in areas with high prevalence [15].

2. Epidemiology of schistosomiasis

2.1 Pathogen agents

Human schistosomiasis is caused by eight species of *Schistosoma*: *S. mansoni* (intestinal schistosomiasis agent), *S. haematobium* (urinary schistosomiasis agent), *S. mattheei* (urinary schistosomiasis agent), *S. guineensis* (rectal schistosomiasis agent), *S. intercalatum* (rectal schistosomiasis agent), *S. japonicum* (arteriovenous schistosomiasis agent), *S. maleyensis* (arteriovenous schistosomiasis agent), and *S. mekongi* (arteriovenous schistosomiasis agent) [16].

The most causes of disease are *S. mansoni* and *S. haematobium*. People are infected when *Schistosomes* are transmitted during contact with freshwater contaminated with human excreta containing parasite eggs. A gastropod host must be present in the water for the parasite to complete its life cycle.

2.2 Simplified *Schistosoma* life cycle

There exist two phases of *Schistosoma* multiplication: the asexual phase in the intermediate host (freshwater mollusks) and the sexual phase in the definitive host (parasitized man) [1].

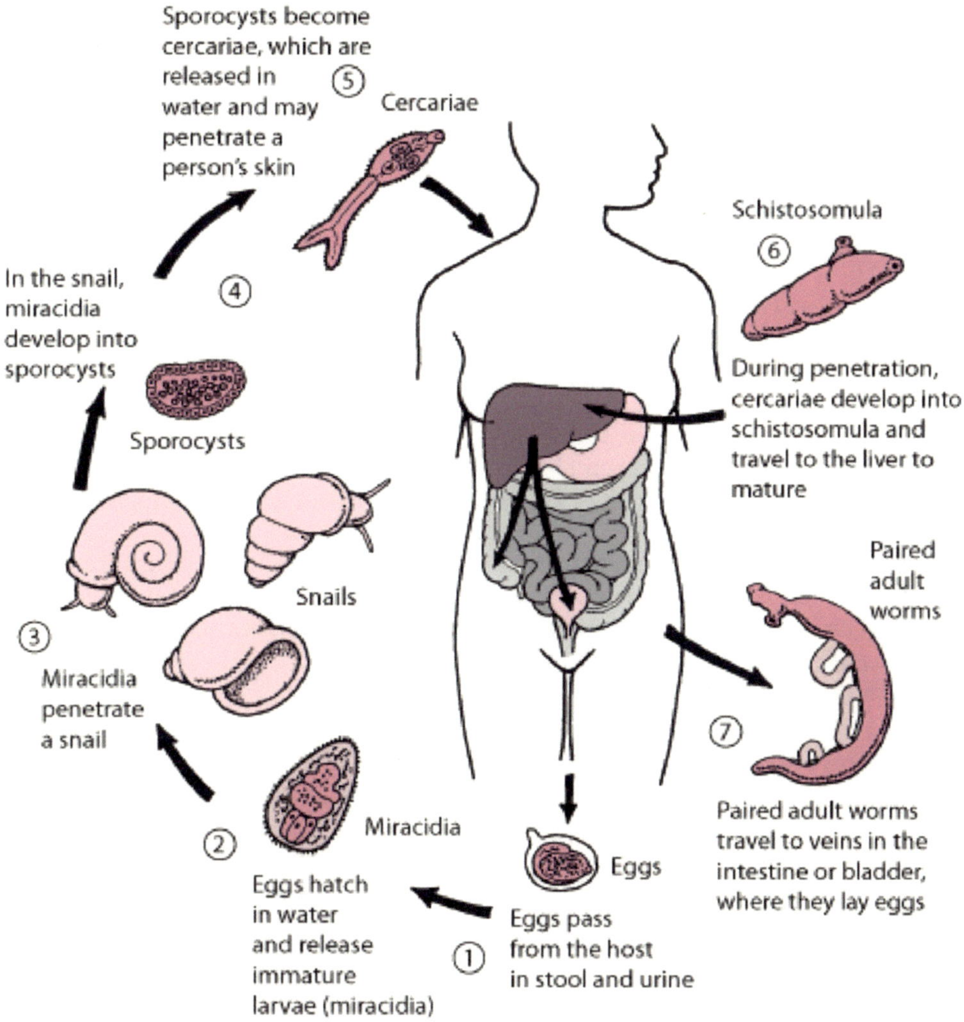

In people, the *Schistosome* eggs are eliminated in feces or urine into water (1). In water, under optimal conditions, the eggs hatch and release immature *Schistosome* larvae called miracidia (2). The miracidia swim and penetrate specific snail intermediate hosts (3). Miracidia evolve into sporocysts within the snail (4) Sporocysts mature into cercaria, which are discharged into the water by the snail and penetrate the skin of the human victim (5). Cercariae lose their tail and become schistosomula when they penetrate the skin. After that, the schistosomula move to the liver to mature into adults. Male and female worms become corpulent and move to intestinal or bladder veins (depending on their species). *S. japonicum*, for example, is found more frequently in the superior mesenteric veins that drain the small intestine, whereas *S. mansoni* is found more frequently in the inferior mesenteric veins that drain the large intestine. Both species, on the other hand, can live in either location and move between them. *S. haematobium* is found in the bladder's vesicular and pelvic venous plexus, as well as the rectal venules. *S. intercalatum* and *S. guineensis* are also found in the inferior mesenteric plexus, but they are located lower in the bowel than *S. mansoni*. There, where they remain, the females begin to lay eggs (7). The eggs are moved progressively toward the lumen of the intestine (*S. mansoni, S. japonicum, S. mekongi, S. intercalatum/guineensis*) and of the bladder and ureters (*S. haematobium*), and are eliminated with feces or urine, respectively.

2.3 Clinical manifestations of schistosomiasis

Human schistosomiasis symptoms are caused by the body's reaction to the parasitic eggs, not by the parasites themselves [1]. Many infections are symptomless. Following cercariae penetration, a cutaneous hypersensitivity reaction might occur, manifesting as tiny, itchy maculopapular sores. Katayama fever is a systemic hypersensitivity reaction caused by *S. japonicum* and *S. mansoni* that can occur weeks after the initial infection. Systemic symptoms such as stomach pain, diarrhea, fever, cough, eosinophilia, and hepatosplenomegaly are among the clinical signs.

Infections with *Schistosoma* can cause lesions in the central nervous system. Ectopic *S. japonicum* eggs in the brain can cause cerebral granulomatous disease, and granulomatous lesions around ectopic eggs in the spinal cord can occur in *S. mansoni* and *S. haematobium* infections. Persistent infection can lead to granulomatous responses and fibrosis in the liver and spleen, as well as other symptoms.

Various hepatic complications from inflammation and granulomatous reactions, as well as embolic egg granulomas in the brain and spinal cord, are associated with *S. mansoni* and *S. japonicum* schistosomiasis. Hematuria, scarring, calcification, squamous cell carcinoma, and embolic egg granulomas in the brain and spinal cord are all symptoms of *S. haematobium* schistosomiasis.

2.4 Reservoirs of *Schistosoma*

Cattle, dogs, cats, rodents, pigs, horses, and goats serve as reservoirs for *S. japonicum*, while dogs serve as reservoirs for *S. mekongi* [1]. In endemic areas, *S. mansoni* is frequently recovered from wild primates, but it is primarily a human parasite rather than a zoonosis.

2.5 *Schistosoma*'s hosts

These parasites develop successively in two hosts: the intermediate host and the definitive host [1]. Intermediate hosts are freshwater snails of the genera *Biomphalaria*, (*S. mansoni*), *Oncomelania* (*S. japonicum*), *Bulinus* (*S. haematobium, S. intercalatum, S. guineensis*). The only known intermediate host for *S. mekongi* is *Neotricula aperta*. The definitive host is usually humans but maybe cattle.

The hatched eggs enter a small aquatic snail, to spend the first part of their life there. Then the eggs become small worms, called cercariae, which swim and contaminate the human host, which is in contact with water, by crossing the skin, entering the veins, then in the digestive tract where the eggs are laid and then eliminated by the stools in the aquatic environment.

2.6 Risk groups

There is no natural immunity in humans. However, the slow development of acquired resistance to reinfection appears with age [1].

The groups most particularly exposed to the risk of schistosomiasis are school-aged children, teenagers, adults belonging to certain professional categories (fishermen, rice farmers), women who come into contact with infested water during their household chores, and entire communities in high-risk areas. The disease can manifest itself in intestinal or urogenital form.

2.7 Risk factors

Schistosomiasis is an important cause of disease in many parts of the world, most commonly in places with poor sanitation [17]. As a result, social-ecological processes control schistosomiasis transmission (e.g., conditions of poverty and living near open freshwater bodies). Humans excrete *Schistosome* eggs in their feces or urine. Miracidia infect particular snails after hatching to produce cercariae. During household (e.g., washing clothes or dishes) and recreational activities, *Schistosome* cercariae penetrate the unbroken skin of humans (e.g., bathing and swimming in unprotected open freshwater bodies).

Living near freshwater bodies (e.g., rivers, small dams, irrigation schemes, and lakes), socioeconomic factors that influence occupational activities (e.g., poor people without running water at home are more likely to contact freshwater bodies), and climate change have all been shown to facilitate schistosomiasis transmission in Africa. The lack of access to proper sanitation encourages open defecation, which pollutes the environment and increases schistosomiasis transmission.

2.8 Geographic distribution

There are many species of *Schistosoma* that are only known for animal infections. Out of the 22 currently recognized species, only eight have been reported from humans and of these, only three are heavily implicated as diseases of public health importance [1].

- *S. sinensium, S. japonicum, S. maleyensis, S. mekongi* are found in East and South-East Asia
- *S. hippopotami* in Africa
- *Orientobilharzia turkstanicum and S. incognitum* in Asia
- *S. mansoni and Sirthenea rodhaini* distributed throughout Africa. *S. mansoni* is in some South American countries (Brazil, Suriname, and Venezuela), and in

Caribbean (Dominican Republic, Guadeloupe, Martinique, and Saint Lucia with sporadic reports in the Arabian Peninsula).

- *S. nasale, S. spindale, and S. indicum* in West and South Asia.

- *S. margrebowiei, S. leiperi, S. mattheei, S. intercalatum, S. haematobium, S. guineensis, S. curassoni, and S. bovis* in Africa. *S. haematobium* is found in areas of the Middle East and a recent focus of ongoing transmission has been identified in Corsica. *S. intercalatum* can be found in parts of Central and West Africa, particularly in the Democratic Republic of the Congo. West Africa is home to *S. guineensis*. In Corsica, France, and certain West African countries, infections with hybrid/introgressed *Schistosoma* (*S. haematobium*, × *S. bovis*, × *S. curassoni*, × *S. mattheei*) have been reported.

3. Prevention and control of schistosomiasis

3.1 Prevention of schistosomiasis

There is no vaccine available but its development is underway. The best way to prevent *Schistosoma* infection is to take the following steps if you are visiting or live in an area where schistosomiasis is transmitted [1]:

- Scrupulously avoid contact with contaminated freshwater by swimming or wading when you are in countries in which schistosomiasis occurs. For prevention, swimming in the ocean and chlorinated swimming pools is safe.

- To avoid scorching, freshwater for bathing should be heated for at least 1 minute to destroy any cercariae, then cooled before bathing. Water that has been stored for at least 1 to 2 days in a storage tank, on the other hand, should be safe to drink without boiling.

- People who are inadvertently exposed to potentially contaminated water (for example, by falling into a river) should dry themselves thoroughly with a towel to try to remove any parasites before they reach the skin.

- Drink safe water. Swallowing contaminated water does not spread schistosomiasis; however, mouth and lip contact with contaminated water could lead to infection. Because water directly from canals, lakes, rivers, streams, or springs could be polluted with a range of infectious organisms, you should either boil it for 1 minute or filter it before consuming it. Any hazardous parasites, bacteria, or viruses will be killed by bringing your water to a rolling boil for at least 1 minute.

- Those who have had contact with potentially contaminated water overseas should see their health care provider after returning from travel to discuss testing.

Preventive chemotherapy has been suggested by the WHO as a morbidity control technique to assist reduce the occurrence, extent, and severity of infection's consequences [12].

While preventive chemotherapy cannot prevent reinfection, it can reduce egg production, reducing the morbidity associated with egg deposition in human tissue [18].

Preventive chemotherapy is given to school-aged children in endemic areas because they are at a higher risk of infection. In areas where the prevalence of infection is at least 10%, preventive treatment should be given to those who are at high risk of infection due to their occupation, such as fishermen, farmers, and irrigation workers, as well as women who may be exposed to infected waters while performing domestic chores. Pregnant and lactating women in these areas should be included in preventive chemotherapy campaigns as well, as they are thought to be at a higher risk of schistosomiasis-related morbidity [1].

3.2 Schistosomiasis control and elimination strategies

In the 1920s, Egypt launched the first mass medication administration campaigns in adults and children, using intravenous tartar emetic, in one of the earliest attempts to control schistosomiasis. Following that, a national program was implemented, which included disease-control techniques such as chemotherapy and/or snail control. The development of safe antibiotics for treating human infections, such as niridazole, metrifonate, oxamniquine, and praziquantel, refocused control methods on chemotherapy [19].

The World Health Assembly produced Resolution 54.19 in 2001, endorsing chemotherapy as the primary option for schistosomiasis management by mass medication administration. By 2010, this resolution set a goal of 75–100% frequent chemotherapy coverage for school-aged children (ages 5–14 years) who are at risk of morbidity [12]. However, as acknowledged at the 65th World Health Assembly in May 2012, this goal was not met [20].

In 2010, over 108 million school-aged children required treatment, with at least 21 million receiving treatment (19%), far short of the resolution's target. This was based on reports from 28 (55%) of the 51 countries where schistosomiasis preventive chemotherapy should have been used [21].

Integrated control of schistosomiasis strategy, combining large-scale preventive chemotherapy, hygiene, improved sanitation, education, provision of potable water, snail control, and environmental modification can lead to interruption of schistosomiasis transmission (elimination). There are five stages to an intensified control program that will result in the abolition of schistosomiasis: [22, 23].

- Morbidity management;
- Abolition as a public health issue;
- Transmission interruption (elimination);
- Post-transmission monitoring; As well as
- Verification of elimination.

As a program progresses from one phase to the next, its objectives should be changed, with scaled-up activities such as appropriate public health interventions (snail control and environmental management, WASH, One Health) and a strong surveillance system in place to achieve the specific goal. It may take a country 13–50 years to achieve transmission interruption after launching the first group of morbidity-control interventions, and this will necessitate many interventions (not just preventive chemotherapy) that are implemented effectively, sustained, and uninterrupted, with strong political commitment and investment.

There is no "one-size-fits-all" intervention scenario that can guarantee the eradication of Schistosoma infection because the disease is epidemiologically distinct throughout its geographical distribution. Transmission dynamics, disease pathology, the occurrence of reservoir hosts, the habitat of intermediate snail hosts, and the age pattern at which individuals acquire and resolve infection, as well as patterns of infection exposure, are all affected by key species and ecological differences. Furthermore, some countries have advanced schistosomiasis control or elimination programs, whereas others have yet to initiate programs based on the recommended strategies. Integration of schistosomiasis control and elimination activities with existing preventive chemotherapy programs to control and eliminate other NTDs should thus be considered. Treatment for schistosomiasis may be coordinated with preventive chemotherapy for lymphatic filariasis, onchocerciasis, soil-transmitted helminthiases, and trachoma during the phases of controlling morbidity and elimination as a public health problem [24–26].

In conclusion, Schistosomiasis control focuses on reducing disease through periodic, large-scale population treatment with praziquantel; a more comprehensive approach including potable water, adequate sanitation, and snail control would also reduce transmission. Mass community-based or school-based treatment with praziquantel, education programs, and molluscicides to reduce snail populations are used to control schistosomiasis in endemic areas.

4. Conclusion

Species of the genus *Schistosoma* are various and widespread across the globe, causing infections in humans as well as in animals. In Africa, the public health burden of schistosomiasis, caused primarily by *S. mansoni, S. haematobium*, and *S. intercalatum/ guineensis*, is enormous. No vaccine is available but the best way to prevent schistosomiasis is to avoid swimming or wading in freshwater, drink safe water and the water used for bathing should be brought to a rolling boil for 1 minute. Schistosomiasis control is based on large-scale treatment of at-risk populations, access to safe water, improved sanitation, hygiene education, and snail control. Praziquantel is the preferred treatment for all types of schistosomiasis. It is efficient, safe, and inexpensive. Monitoring is essential to determine the impact of control interventions.

DOI: http://dx.doi.org/10.5772/intechopen.105170

Author details

Célestin Kyambikwa Bisangamo
Institut Supérieur des Techniques Médicales (ISTM-Bukavu), Bukavu,
Democratic Republic of the Congo

*Address all correspondence to: cele.kyambis@gmail.com

References

[1] Centers for Disease Control and Prevention (CDC). Schistosomiasis Infection [Internet]. 2019. Available from: https://www.cdc.gov/dpdx/schistosomiasis/index.html

[2] Word Health Organization (WHO). EMRO. Schistosomiasis - Health Topics [Internet]. 2019. Available from: http://www.emro.who.int/health-topics/

[3] Word Health Organization (WHO). Schistosomiasis: Information for Patients and the General Public [Internet]. 2020. Available from: https://www.cismef.org/page/detail/fr/MSH_D_012552

[4] Hotez PJ, Alvarado M, Basáñez MG, Bolliger I, Bourne R, Boussinesq M, et al. The global burden of disease study 2010: Interpretation and implications for the neglected tropical diseases. PLoS Neglected Tropical Diseases. 2014;**8**(7):e2865

[5] Word Health Organization (WHO). Schistosomiasis [Internet]. 2018. Available from: https://www.who.int/schistosomiasis/en/

[6] Hotez P. Forgotten people, forgotten diseases: The neglected tropical diseases and their impact on global health and development. Emerging Infectious Diseases. 2009;**15**:5101

[7] Colley DG, Bustinduy AL, Secor WEKC. Human schistosomiasis. Lancet (London, England). 2014;**383**(22):53-64

[8] Genital Manifestations of Schistosomiasis. Geneva: World Health Organization; 2018. Available from: https://www.who.int/schistosomiasis/genital_schistosomiasis/en/ [Google Scholar]

[9] Montresor A, Engels D, Ramsan M, Foum ASL. Field test of the 'dose pole' for praziquantel in Zanzibar. Transactions of the Royal Society of Tropical Medicine and Hygiene. 2002;**96**(32):3-4

[10] Montresor A, Crompton DWT, Gyorkos TW, Savioli L. Helminth Control in School-Age Children: A Guide for Managers of Control Programmes. Geneva: World Health Organization; 2002

[11] Webster JP, Molyneux DH, Hotez PJFA. The contribution of mass drug administration to global health: Past, present and future. Philosopical Transactions of the Royal Society of London B Biological Sciences. 2014;**369**:20130434

[12] World Health Organization. Progress Report 2001-2011 and Strategic Plan 2012-2020. Geneva, Switzerland: WHO; 2012

[13] Stothard JR, Campbell SJ, Osei-Atweneboana MY, Durant T, Stanton MC, Biritwum NK, et al. Towards interruption of schistosomiasis transmission in sub-Saharan Africa: Developing an appropriate environmental surveillance framework to guide and to support 'end game'interventions. Infectious Diseases of Poverty. 2017;**6**(1):1-11

[14] Word Health Organization (WHO). Accelerating Work to Overcome the Global Impact of Neglected Tropical Diseases: A Roadmap for Implementation. Geneva: WHO; 2012

[15] Toor J, Alsallaq R, Truscott JE, Turner HC, Werkman M, Gurarie D, et al. Are we on our way to achieving the 2020 goals for schistosomiasis

morbidity control using current World Health Organization guidelines? Clinical Infectious Diseases. 2018;**66**(suppl_4):S245-S252

[16] Record WE. Weekly epidemiological Record, 2019, vol. 94, 50 [full issue]. Weekly Epidemiological Record= Relevé épidémiologique hebdomadaire. 2019;**94**(50):601-612

[17] Angora EK, Boissier J, Menan H, Rey O, Tuo K, Touré AO, et al. Prevalence and risk factors for schistosomiasis among schoolchildren in two settings of Côte d'Ivoire. Tropical Medicine and Infectious Disease. 2019;**4**(3):110

[18] Montgomery S. Schistosomiasis. In: CDC Yellow Book 2020: Health Information for International Travel. Centers for Disease Control and Prevention. Oxford University Press; 2019

[19] Inobaya MT, Olveda RM, Chau TN, Olveda DURA. Prevention and control of schistosomiasis: A current perspective. Reseach and Report in Tropical Medicine. 2014;**5**:65

[20] Word Health Organization (WHO). Schistosomiasis: Number of people treated in 2012. Weekly Epidemiological Record. 2014;**89**(4):21-28

[21] Word Health Organization (WHO). Schistosomiasis: Number of people treated in 2010. Weekly Epidemiological Record. 2012;**87**(4):37-44

[22] Wang LD, Chen HG, Guo JG, Zeng XJ, Hong XL, Xiong JJ, et al. A strategy to control transmission of Schistosoma japonicum in China. The New England Journal of Medicine. 2009;**360**(2):121-128

[23] Kajihara N, Hirayama K. The war against a regional disease in Japan a history of the eradication of schistosomiasis japonica. Tropical Medicine and Health. 2011;**39** (1 Suppl 1):3

[24] Deol A, Fleming F, Calvo-Urbano B, Walker M, Bucumi V, Gnandou I, et al. Schistosomiasis – Assessing progress towards the 2020 and 2025 goals. The New England Journal of Medicine. 2019;**381**(26):2519-2528. DOI: 10.1056/NEJMoa1812165

[25] WHO: Schistosomiasis: Progress Report 2001-2011 and Strategic Plan 2012-2020. Geneva: World Health Organization; 2012 Available from: https://apps.who.int/iris/handle/10665/78074 [Accessed: March 8, 2022]

[26] Khieu V, Sayasone S, Muth S, Kirinoki M, Laymanivong S, Ohmae H, et al. Elimination of schistosomiasis mekongi from endemic areas in Cambodia and the Lao People's Democratic Republic: Current status and plans. Tropical Medicine and Infectious Disease. 2019;**4**(1):30. DOI: 10.3390/tropicalmed4010030

Chapter 3

Schistosoma Mansoni Infection and Therapeutic Efficacy of Praziquantel in Preschool-Aged Children

Genanew Birhanu

Abstract

Schistosomiasis is one of the extreme scientific results which can be greater usual in sub-Saharan Africa. It impacts growth, bodily fitness, and cognitive function, mainly in children. The maximum not unusual place method to manipulate schistosomiasis is preventive chemotherapy. Though World Health Organization (WHO) recommends praziquantel for the manage and remedy of schistosomiasis, preschool-aged children (PSAC) are excluded from populace remedy applications specifically due to paucity of statistics on reaction rate. The findings of preceding research accomplished to evaluate the impact of chemotherapy on schistosomiasis confirmed a few variation. This indicates the need for in addition research in one of the kind populations.

Keywords: *Schistosoma mansoni*, Praziquantel, therapeutic efficacy, preschool children

1. Introduction

1.1 Background

Schistosomiasis is a sickness resulting from parasitic flatworms of the genus Schistosoma. Clinical schistosomiasis is primarily associated with symptoms that include dizziness, abdominal pain, nausea, vomiting, mild diarrhea, fever, and toxic or allergic reactions. In some cases, however, the disease can evolve to life-threatening complications and causes a wide range of mortality [1]. There are around over 229 million people currently require preventive treatment against this disease, the vast majority of who live in sub-Saharan Africa [2]. In 2017, an predicted 1.4 million incapacity-adjusted existence years (DALYs) had been misplaced to schistosomiasis, accounting for 8.3% of the entire sickness burden resulting from the neglected tropical diseases (NTDs) [1, 3].

Preventive chemotherapy is the number one worldwide method for controlling the morbidity due to schistosomiasis. It is the periodic control of single-dose oral praziquantel (usually given at 40 mg/kg body weight), in which praziquantel is administered without preceding analysis to complete companies or aim companies, most importantly faculty-aged children, counting on the volume of endemicity [4]. The goal is to reduce diease morbidity and transmission toward the removal of the diseases as a public fitness problem. Periodic treatment of at-risk population will cure mild sympthoms and prevent infected people from developing severe, late-stage chronic diseases [5, 6].

However preschool-aged children (PSAC), who are individuals below the age of 5 years, are currently excluded from preventive chemotherapy control campaigns. However, current research finished in exclusive elements of East and West Africa confirmed that during excessive endemicity regions, a good sized percentage of PSAC is already inflamed with *Schistosoma spp.*, and subsequently remedy would possibly want to be prolonged to more youthful age companies in such excessive chance regions [7, 8].

1.2 Statement of the problem

The World Health Organization (WHO) introduced a road map to combat NTDs by 2030; the plan was introduced in 2012 and the goal is to reduce the prevalence of moderate and heavy infections with schistosomiasis, so it become no longer public health problems. By considering this, Ethiopia also set a similar goal to achieve the same goal by the same year using different control measures like periodic mass administration of preventive chemotherapy (deworming) [9, 10].

WHO recommending regular de-worming of SAC (school age children, 5–14 years) and adults (>15 years old) who reside within disease endemic regions and at risk of infection with antihelminthic [9–11]. On the other hand, studies have also revealed that children aged 5 years and below can be commonly infected by shistosomiasis [12, 13]. Therefore for some, their disease-related morbidity and discomfort have not been averted as quickly or as successfully as possible [14].

Until recently, the parasitological overall performance of praziquantel withinside the more youthful youngster was not nicely known, cooccurring with the general loss of formal documentation and pharmacological medicinal drug of this drug in its use in toddlers and PSAC [15]. Hence, PSAC mostly share similar risk of schistosomiasis with adults that have an effect on normal deworming at the epidemiology and route of schistosomiasis merits extra attention to evaluate the effect of interventions, the adequacy of techniques implemented, and the development made withinside the combat toward anemia. It is likewise vital to set included manipulate packages and compare the effectiveness of manipulate interventions [16]. The initial outcomes of pilot research confirmed that remedy with praziquantel is secure and efficacious on this age institution for the remedy of schistosomiasis [16, 17]. But the state of affairs in regions endemic for schistosomiasis like Ethiopia is unknown [17].

Younger kids are predisposed to heavy infections with intestinal parasites due to the fact their immune structures are not but completely developed, and in addition they habitually play in fecally infected soil [18]. A look carried out in Uganda suggests that 42.1% of PSAC had detectable *S. mansoni* egg [19]. The incidence of *S. mansoni* in PSAC became 25.5% in AzaguieMakouguie and 21.6% in AzaguieM'Bromedistrics of Ivory Coast [20].

There is developing recognition that during excessive endemicity settings, schistosomiasis is likewise not an unusual place in PSAC, and as a result those younger kids may want to be covered in deworming campaigns [21].

DOI: http://dx.doi.org/10.5772/intechopen.103901

Research is likewise had to correctly decide the protection, frequency, and severity of unfavorable occasions after praziquantel management toward schistosomiasis withinside the preschool-aged population [20, 22]. According to a minimum reproduction Kato-Katz thick smears, 35 PSAC of per-protocol population (21.9%) had been determined S. mansoni-positive [22]. Study carried out in Wondo Genet; South Ethiopia exhibits that 85.1% of children under the age of five youngsters had been determined to be inflamed with one or extra intestinal parasites, the superiority of *S. mansoni* rank second subsequent to *Trichuristrichiura* constituting 37.2% [23, 24].

In Ethiopia, numerous research assessed the significance of occurrence schistosomiasis among school youngsters [25, 26]. Only few research have suggested the significance of intestinal parasitic infections among beneathneath 5 youngsters [23]. But the suggested findings at the protection of praziquantel in preschool-aged youngsters as preventive chemotherapy for schistosomiasis is not always indicated clearly [10].

Although praziquantel now no longer used as a mass preventive chemotherapy for PSAC for the motive of paucity of records at the efficacy and protection on this age group, it is getting used as first-line remedy for beneathneath 5 medical case of schistosomiasis [27]. To add evidence on the usage of PZQ, this have a look at to evaluate the healing efficacy and protection of praziquantel in PSAC (<5 years) in a place in which *S. mansoni* endemic in SAC.

2. Literature review

Schistosomias is public health problem which mainly affects developing countries with major consequences for human health as well as social and economic development. It occurs at all stages of the life, but it is more prevalent in pregnant women and young children. It is a critical health concern, since it affects growth and energy level adversely. Globally, schistosomias affects around 200 million people. Most of them are PSAC and school age children in developing countries [28–31].

Moderate and intense schistosomia depth is related to persistent unfavorable results on nutrition A and iron status, physical, intellectual, and cognitive improvement specifically in youngsters, those morbidities which take a big effect at the fitness of youngsters [22, 32, 33]. Also the geographical distribution of PSAC is basically restrained to the zones wherein fashionable ailment transmission may be very high, for example, in regions wherein pre-national disease control programs (NDCP) occurrence in SAC is nicely greater than over 50% [14].

There are two major reasons why schistosomiasis is one of the public health problems in infants and PSAC. First, this young age group plays a great role in helping to maintain local disease transmission, even though these infected children may be excreting fewer eggs. Besides, rinsing and washing children's soiled clothes in environmental water bodies also contribute toward more cryptic contamination and disease transmission [15, 27, 29].

The second viable cause entails ordinary water contact. That stops the infection related with water and multiplied re-contamination episodes, which additionally ends in a modern boom of person bug burden. It is consequently in all likelihood that untreated infections received in early youth make contributions to worsening the longer time period medical image of the sickness withinside the person [14]. The anthelmintic drug praziquantel is the cornerstone for morbidity management because of schistosomiasis [14]. Emphasis is positioned on SAC, while PSAC (people underneath the age of 5 years) are generally excluded from preventive chemotherapy.

However, in exceedingly endemic areas, a large amount of PSAC is already stricken by schistosomiasis [29]. For that cause, there is an ongoing dialog whether or not preventive chemotherapy with praziquantel ought to be prolonged to preschoolers [17, 29].

Previous findings confirmed that beaten praziquantel (forty mg/kg) administered to PSAC is quite efficacious with cure rates (CRs) around 90% and egg discount rate (ERR) above 95%, while preferred diagnostic methods (Kato-Katz for *S. mansoni* and urine filtration for *S. haematobium*) had been used and furnished new perception into the efficacy and protection of praziquantel among a ignored populace organization in a *S. mansoni* and *S. haematobium* co-endemic location [22].

The latest examine accomplished in PSAC in Uganda, the usage of quadruplicate Kato-Katz thick smears, mentioned a barely decrease efficacy of praziquantel in opposition to *S. mansoni* (CR, 80.2%; ERR, 87.9%) [14]. Another examine performed withinside the identical location mentioned big concern findings as the general CR among 305 *S. mansoni* egg patent people changed into simplest 56.4%, with especially low CR found in preschoolers with a records of preceding praziquantel treatments (CR 41.7%) [17]. PSAC in co-endemic districts of well-known Ivoire Coast shows excessive efficacy in opposition to *S. mansoni* (CR, 88.6%; ERR, 96.7%) [22].

WHO advocates mass treatment at colleges with the frequency of treatment obsessed with prevalence, and intensity of shistosomiasis infection, but with magnified prevalence through irrigation, ponds and dynamic water bodies, and different at-risk populations might have to be enclosed in treatment programs [34]. In September 2010, an off-the-cuff 2-day meeting came about in Geneva that brought along new proof from many countries regarding the prevalence of schistosomiasis within the younger kid also because of the performance of praziquantel treatment for encouraging changes in its formal licensing or off-label use in treatment of young kids [35].

Studies conducted in five African countries with high prevalence of schistosomiasis (n = 3198) reported high CR, and significant reductions in mean egg counts occurred for both urogenital and intestinal schistosomiasis [32]. Recently, a report showed that praziquantel alone and in combination with mebendazole in the treatment of *S. mansoni* and soil-transmitted helminthes in PSAC showed similar safety profiles [36, 37].

Treatment of youngsters with praziquantel is ethically warranted, is tried to be safe, and may be enforced with success on the bottom within the frame of preventive chemotherapy. This means the necessity of progressive scale-up of management at the national level. If the above steps are taken and pharmacokinetic studies assist to more optimize pragmatic dosing, praziquantel treatment gap might be closed within the predictable future. By giving infants and PSAC access to medication, this could cause real progress in the management of pediatric infection in the public health setting [21, 32].

3. Conclusion

The prevalence of intestinal schistosomiasis could be very hign in preschool-aged children which really showes a major public health problem. Children with the age of five have been much likely affected with the infection of *S. mansoni* in comparision with children less than 5 years of age. Administering crushed praziquantel at a dose of 40 mg/kg showed good therapeutic efficacy for *S. mansoni* in preschool-aged children.

Abbrevations/acronyms

CR	Cure rate
ERR	Egg reduction rate
EPG	Eggs per gram
NTD	Neglected tropical disease
PSAC	Preschool-aged children
SAC	School age children
WHO	World Health Organization

Author details

Genanew Birhanu
Department of Medical Laboratory Science, College of Medicine and Health Sciences, Arba Minch University, Arba Minch, Ethiopia

*Address all correspondence to: birhanufasil13@gmail.com

References

[1] Worku L, Damte D, Endris M, Tesfa H, Aemero M. *Schistosoma mansoni* infection and associated determinant factors among school children in Sanja town, Northwest Ethiopia. Journal of Parasitology Research. 2014:792536

[2] WHO. Schistosomiasis: Fact Sheet. 2020a. Accessed from: https://www.who.int/news-room/fact-sheets/detail/schistosomiasis [Accessed: July 15, 2020]

[3] DALYs, HALE Collaborators. Global, regional, and national disability-adjusted lifeyears (DALYs) for 359 diseases and injuries and healthy life expectancy (HALE) for 195 countries and territories, 1990-2017: A systematic analysis for the global burden of disease study 2017. Lancet. 2018;**392**(10159):1859-1922. [Accessed: November 10, 2018]

[4] WHO. Assessing the Efficacy of Anthelminthic Drugs against Schistosomiasis and Soil- Transmitted Helminthiases. Geneva: World Health Organization; 2013b

[5] Carter Center. Schistosomiasis Control Program. Nigeria: Carter Center; 2015. Available from: www.cartercenter.org [Accessed: August 2015]

[6] Fenwick A, Savioli L, Engels D, Bergquist NR, Todd MH. Drugs for the control of parasitic diseases: Current status and development in schistosomiasis. Trends in Parasitology. 2003;**19**:509-515

[7] Mafiana CF, Ekpo UF, Ojo DA. Urinary schistosomiasis in preschool children in settlements around Oyan reservoir in Ogun state, Nigeria: Implications for control. Tropical Medicine & International Health. 2003;**8**:78-82

[8] Garba A, Barkire N, Djibo A, et al. Schistosomiasis in infants and preschool-aged children: Infection in a single *S. haematobium* and a mixed *S. haematobium-S. mansoni* foci of Niger. Acta Tropica. 2010;**115**:212-219

[9] WHO. The World Health Assembly Resolution (WHA 54.19). Geneva: World Health Organization; 2001. Available from: http://www.who.int/inf-pr-2001/en/pr2001WHA-6.html [Accessed: November 20, 2015]

[10] Anthony D, Aragon, Reza A, et al. Towards an understanding of the mechanism of action of praziquantel. Molecular and Biochemical Parasitology. 2010;**164**:58-63

[11] Fenwick A, Webster JP, Bosque-Oliva E, et al. The schistosomiasis control initiative (SCI): Rationale, development and implementation from 2002-2008. Parasitology. 2009;**136**(1719-1730):27

[12] Bosompem KM, Bentum IA, Otchere J, et al. Infant schistosomiasis in Ghana: A survey in an irrigation community. Tropical Medicine & International Health. 2004;**9**:917-922

[13] Odogwu SE, Ramamurthy NK, Kabatereine N, et al. Schistosoma mansoni in infants (aged <3 years) along the Ugandan shoreline of (Lake Victoria <3 years) along the Ugandan shoreline of Lake Victoria. Annals of Tropical Medicine and Parasitology. 2006;**100**:315-326

[14] Stothard JR, Sousa-Figueiredo JC, Betson M, et al. Closing the praziquantel treatment gap: New steps in epidemiological monitoring and control of schistosomiasis in African infants and

preschool-aged children. Parasitology. 2011;**138**:1593-1606

[15] Stothard JR, Gabrielli AF. Schistosomiasis in African infants and preschool children: To treat or not to treat? Trends in Parasitology. 2007;**23**:83-86

[16] WHO. Investing to overcome the global impact of neglected tropical diseases. In: Third Who Report on Neglected Tropical Diseases? Geneva, Switzerland: WHO Document Production Services; 2015

[17] Sousa-Figueiredo JC, Betson M, Atuhaire A, et al. Performance and safety of praziquantel for treatment of intestinal schistosomiasis in infants and preschool children. PLoS Neglected Tropical Diseases. 2012;**6**:e1864

[18] Rao V, Sugunan A, Murhekar M, Sehgal S. Malnutrition and high childhood mortality among the Onge tribe of the Andaman and Nicobar Islands. Public Health Nutrition. 2006;**9**:19-25

[19] De Moira AP, Sousa-Figueiredo JC, Jones FM, et al. *S. mansoni* infection in preschool-aged children: Development of immunoglobulin E and immunoglobulin G4 responses to parasite allergen-like proteins. Journal of Infectious Diseases. 2012;**207**:302-306

[20] Coulibaly JT. Epidemiology and Diagnosis of Schistosomiasis in Preschool-Aged Children in Azaguié, South Côte d'Ivoire. Côte d'Ivoire: Coulibaly JT; 2013. Unpublished

[21] Sousa-Figueiredo JC, Pleasant J, Day M, et al. Treatment of intestinal schistosomiasis in Ugandan preschool children: Best diagnosis, treatment efficacy and side-effects, and an extended praziquantel dosing pole. International Health. 2010;**2**:103-113

[22] Mutamad A, Mohamed S, Mohamed K, et al. Treatment of pre-school children under 6 years of age for schistosomiasis: Safety, efficacy and acceptability of praziquantel. Sudan JMS. 2012;**7**(2):28

[23] Coulibaly JT, N'Gbesso YK, Knopp S, et al. Efficacy and safety of Praziquantel in preschool-aged children in an area Co-endemic for *S. mansoni* and *S. haematobium*. PLoS Neglected Tropica Diseases. 2012;**6**(12):e1917

[24] Nyantekyi AL, Legesse M, Belay M, et al. Intestinal parasitic infections among under-five children and maternal awareness about the infections in Sheshamane Kebele, Wondo genet, southern Ethiopia. Ethiopian Journal of Health Development. 2010;**24**(3):186-190

[25] Ayalew A, Debebe T, Worku A. Prevalence and risk factors of intestinal parasites among Delgi school children, North Gondar, Ethiopia. Journal of Parasitology and Vector Biology. 2011;**3**(5):75-81

[26] Erko B, Medhin G. Human helminthiasis in Wondo genet, southern Ethiopia, with emphasis on geo-helminthiasis. Ethiopian Medical Journal. 2003;**41**:333-344

[27] Mutapi F, Rujeni N, Bourke C, et al. Schistosoma haematobium treatment in 1-5 year old children: Safety and efficacy of the antihelminthic drug praziquantel. PLoS Neglected Tropica Diseased. 2011;**5**:e1143

[28] King CH, Dickman K, Tisch DJ. Reassessment of the cost of chronic helminthic infection: A meta-analysis of disability-related outcomes in endemic schistosomiasis. Lancet. 2005;**365**:1561-1569

[29] Gryseels B, Polman K, Clerinx J, Kestens L. Human schistosomiasis. Lancet. 2006;**368**:1106-1118

[30] Utzinger J, Raso G, Brooker S, et al. Schistosomiasis and neglected tropical diseases: Towards integrated and sustainable control and a word of caution. Parasitology. 2009;**136**:1859-1874

[31] Steinmann P, Keiser J, Bos R, Tanner M, Utzinger J. Schistosomiasis and water resources development: Systematic review, meta-analysis, and estimates of people at risk. The Lancet Infectious Diseases. 2006;**6**:411-425

[32] Gray DJ, Ross AG, Li YS, McManus DP. Diagnosis and management of schistosomiasis. BMJ. 2011;**342**:d2651

[33] WHO. Report of a Meeting to Review the Results of Studies on the Treatment of Schistosomiasis in Preschool-Age Children. Geneva, Switzerland: WHO Document Production Services; 2011

[34] Myra T. Global trends in schistosomiasis control. Department of Community Health, University of Kwa Zulu-Natal, Durban, South Africa. Bulletin of the World Health Organization. 2008;**86**(10). DOI: 10.2471/BLT.08.058669

[35] Keiser J, Ingram K, Utzinger J. Antiparasitic drugs for paediatrics: Systematic review, formulations, pharmacokinetics, safety, efficacy and implications for control. Parasitology. 2011;**138**:1620-1632

[36] Utzinger J, Keiser J. Schistosomiasis and soil-transmitted helminthiasis: Common drugs for treatment and control. Expert Opinion on Pharmacotherapy. 2004;**5**:263-285

[37] Namwanje H, Kabatereine NB, Olsen A. The acceptability and safety of praziquantel alone and in combination with mebendazole in the treatment of Schistosoma mansoni and soil-transmitted helminthiasis in children aged 1-4 years in Uganda. Parasitology. 2011;**138**:1586-1592

Chapter 4

Treatment Failure, Knowledge, Attitude and Practices Related to Schistosomiasis and Soil-Transmitted Helminthic Infections among Basic School Pupils

Benjamin Amoani, Gideon Kwesi Nakotey, Samuel Asamoah Sakyi, Karen Pomeyie and Christian Sewor

Abstract

Soil-transmitted helminth (STH) and Schistosomiasis infections remain prevalent in developing countries. In Ghana, periodic mass drug administration (MDA) exercise has been implemented to tackle these infections, however, information on drug treatment failure and knowledge of the infection trend is needed for evaluating and modifying existing control programs. This study assessed the knowledge, attitude and practices (KAP) that predispose Basic School pupils to Schistosomiasis and soil-transmitted helminth infections and determined the rate of treatment failure against the worms after school mass drug administration (MDA). A cross-sectional study with a structured questionnaire was used to obtain information on the KAP among pupils who had undergone a MDA (albendazole and praziquantel) exercise 21 days prior. A majority of the pupils interviewed had knowledge of helminthiasis. There were significant associations between helminthic infection and source of drinking water (river; $p = 0.013$), the number of individuals who share toilet facilities ($p = 0.049$) and garbage disposal into a river ($p = 0.015$). Treatment failure of 7.2% was recorded for all the helminthic infections. Potential drug treatment failure of albendazole against hookworm infection and praziquantel against Schistosomiasis infection was thus evident within the population.

Keywords: treatment failure, knowledge, attitude, mass drug administration, soil-transmitted helminths and schistosomiasis

1. Introduction

Soil-transmitted helminthic (STH) infections present a great and silent burden of morbidity and mortality especially in poor populations [1]. It is estimated that STH infections affect more than two billion people worldwide, with the highest prevalence occurring in sub-Saharan Africa, the Americas, China, and East Asia [2]. Helminthic infections are caused by worms such as *Ancylostoma duodenale*, *Necator americanus*, *Ascaris lumbricoides*, *Trichuris trichiura,* and schistosomes. Predominantly, their mode of transmission is through the ingestion of eggs from food contaminated with human faeces that harbour the eggs of the parasite [3]. STH infections have been observed to be prevalent among people living in rural or deprived urban areas with low socio-economic status, lack of potable water, and poor sanitation with children, pregnant women, and farmers who come into contact with the soil regularly being the populations most at risk [4]. STH infections are often associated with intestinal damage which results in nutritional loss thus causing poor mental and physical development and anaemia [5, 6]. These pathologies often lead to a low tolerance to other infections in infants, as well as poor birth outcomes in pregnant women [5].

In addressing morbidity and mortality associated with STH infections WHO has recommended the adoption of monitoring and preventive strategies such as promotion of WASH practices like personal hygiene, proper handling of sewage, and improving the quality of water supply [7]. This is also supplemented with periodic mass administration of antihelminthic drugs such as albendazole and praziquantel via school-based recovery services [7–9].

In Ghana, owing to the high prevalence of STH and Schistosomiasis infections often due to poor sanitary conditions, the country has for the past decades implemented various control measures such as intermittent health education and deworming programs particularly for school children in helminth endemic areas [5, 10–12]. This however has not been complemented with research to monitor the effectiveness of these programs. It is thus against this background that this study was undertaken to assess the rate of treatment failure, knowledge, attitude, and practice of Basic school pupils towards STH and Schistosomiasis infections. The findings from this study highlight an issue of treatment failure. Therefore, this study serves as a wake-up call to the Ministry of Health about the possible need for a mob up exercise. The research also emphasises the need to promote effective control measures towards the eradication of helminthic infections in Ghana.

2. Methodology

2.1 Study design and site

This was a cross-sectional study conducted in Assin Manso within the Central Region of Ghana. It is located 40 kilometres along the Cape Coast– Kumasi highway. Most of the inhabitants are persistent farmers. The study was conducted among Assin Manso A and B Community Basic Schools pupils in the Assin South District, Ghana.

2.2 Study population and sample size

A total of one hundred and fifty-five (155) pupils from kindergarten to Junior High School who had received Praziquantel and albendazole during MDA exercises were randomly selected to participate in the study. The study excluded all pupils who did not participate in the MDA exercise. Participants in this study were strictly pupils within the age range of 5 to 20 years who reside and attend school at Assin Manso Community Basic Schools (A&B).

2.3 Data collection

A structured questionnaire was used to collect data on the knowledge, attitude, and practices of the pupils. This was assessed by asking participants about the signs and symptoms, causes, mode of transmission, prevention, and treatment of helminthic infections. Participant sociodemographic data comprising of age, gender, level of education, occupation of parents, environmental factors concerning potable water, number of water bodies used in the locality and the history of helminthic infections were also collected. Before the commencement of the data collection process, the details of the research were explained to both parents and pupils before questionnaires were administered. The questionnaires were solely developed in clear English language.

Clean stool and urine containers were given to the students to collect stool and urine samples for the parasitological examination. A total of 153 students presented their samples to be used for the parasitological analysis to detect the presence of eggs and worms post Mass Drug Administration (MDA). The urine samples were taken between the hours of 10:00 am and 2:00 pm since this is the appropriate time for optimum egg shedding for *Schistosoma sp.* It was ensured that stool and urine samples were taken to the laboratory at the Department of Biomedical Sciences and kept in a fridge at a temperature of 4°C until ready for the analysis.

2.4 Urine analysis

About 10 mL of the urine sample were transferred into 15 ml falcon tubes and centrifuged at 1500 rpm for 5 minutes. The supernatants were discarded and the sediments were placed on a glass slide. The slides were covered with a coverslip and viewed under an X10 objective lens and X40 upon observation of a likely helminthic egg.

2.5 Saline preparation method

A few drops of saline were added to a little amount of stool in a container and the solution was mixed. Few drops of the resulting solution were placed on a glass slide and covered with a coverslip. The slide was observed under a microscope using the low power X10 objective lens. Upon observation of a suspicious helminthic egg, the X40 objective lens was used for clearer identification.

2.6 Formalin-ether concentration

A wooden stick was used to pick 1gram of stool into a beaker containing 10 ml of 10% formalin and emulsified it into suspension. The suspension was strained through a double layer of wet gauze directly into a 15 ml centrifuge tube. The gauze was discarded, and the suspension in the tube was topped up with formalin to bring the total volume to 7 ml. 3 ml of ether was added to obtain a total volume of 10 ml and the suspension was shaken vigorously. The mixture was centrifuged at 1200xg for 5 minutes. The supernatant was decanted and a few drops of residual fluid was allowed to flow back unto the sediment. A few drops of physiological saline were added to the sediment and re-suspended to have enough fluid. A few drops of the suspension were transferred onto a microscope slide, covered with a coverslip and examined using the low power (X10) objective. The X40 objective was used upon observation of an organism or suspicious objects for detailed morphological examination/identification of the organism.

2.7 Ethical consideration

Ethical clearance was obtained from the Ministry of Education and Scientific Review Committee of the University of Cape Coast. The assent of the parents and teachers were also sought before samples were taken from the pupils for the study.

2.8 Statistical analysis

Data analysis was performed using IBM SPSS Version 26. The distribution of study participants characteristics and prevalence of helminthic infections were presented as frequencies. Chi-square analysis was used to assess the association between study participant characteristics and helminthic status. A p-value <0.05 was considered statistically significant.

3. Results

3.1 Demographic information

The demographic and background characteristics of the study participants are presented in **Table 1**. More than half (57.4%) of the study participants were females and the majority (61.9%) of the study participants were within the age group of 10–14 years. Students in lower primary constituted the majority (31%) of the study participant followed by upper primary (28.6%) then, junior high school (27.4%) with the least being kindergarten students (11.9%). The majority (48.4%) of the study participants' parents are farmers followed by small scale traders (16.1%).

3.2 Knowledge and self-reported symptoms associated with Schistosomiasis and Soil-transmitted helminthic infections

The knowledge and self-reported symptoms associated with schistosomiasis and soil-transmitted helminthic infections of the study participants are presented in **Table 2**. Out of the 155 study participants interviewed, more than half (63.9%) had not heard of helminthiasis, with only 32% being knowledgeable of helminthic infection. However, 45.2% of the participants thought personal hygiene is needed to fight against helminthiasis while (25.8%) did not know if personal hygiene affects helminthiasis or not. 36.1%, 6.5%.6.5%, 3.2%, and 1.3% of the study population said they experienced abdominal pain, diarrhoea, vomiting, pain when urinating (dysuria) and blood in the urine (hematuria) respectively.

3.3 Domestic attitudes related to schistosomiasis and soil-transmitted helminthic infections

Attitudinal characteristics of study participants are presented in **Table 3**. Of all the participants the data shows that the majority (45.2%), (31.1%), (43.2%) of the study

Characteristics	Total (n = 155), n (%)
Gender	
Males	66(42.6)
Females	89(57.4)
Age group (years)	
5–9	42(27.1)
10–14	96(61.9)
15–19	17(11.0)
Level of Education	
Kindergarten	10(11.9)
Lower primary	26(31.0)
Upper primary	24(28.6)
Junior High School	23(27.4)
Occupation of parents	
Farmer	93(60)
Small trader	25(16.1)
Tailor/seamstress	10(6.5)
Mason	5(3.2)
Driver	12(7.7)
Hairdresser	3(1.9)
Mechanic	5(3.2)
Others	2(1.3)

Table 1.
Demographic and background characteristics of study participants.

Characteristics	Total (n = 155), n (%)	
Do you know about helminthiasis		
Yes	56 (36.1)	
No	99 (63.9)	
Do you know how to get a helminthic infection		
Yes	49 (32.0)	
No	72 (47.1)	
Do not know	32 (20.9)	
Is personal hygiene needed to fight helminthiasis		
Yes	70(45.2)	
No	45(29)	
Do not know	40(25.8)	
Symptoms and Experiences	**Yes**	**No**
Do you experience abdominal pain	41(36.1)	114(73.5)

Characteristics	Total (n = 155), n (%)	
Do you experience Diarrhoea	10(6.5)	145(93.5)
Do you experience vomiting	10(.5)	145(93.5)
Do you experience pain when urinating	5(3.2)	150(96.8)
Do you experience blood in the urine	2(1.3)	153(98.7)

Table 2.
Knowledge and self-reported symptoms associated with schistosomiasis and soil-transmitted helminthic infections.

Characteristics	Total (n = 155), n (%)	Total (n = 155), n (%)
Source of water for drinking	**Yes**	**No**
Pipe water	70(45.2)	85(54.8)
Borehole	21(13.5)	134(86.5)
Rainwater	11(7.1)	144(92.9)
Dam	0(0)	155(100)
River water	56(36.1)	99(63.9)
Pond/lake	3(1.9)	152(98.1)
Well	2(1.3)	153(98.7)
Spring	2(1.3)	153(98.7)
Sources of Water for Bathing		
Pipe water	49(31.6)	106(68.4)
Borehole	21(13.5)	134(86.5)
Rainwater	8(5.2)	147(94.8)
Dam	0(0.00)	155(100)
River water	56(36.1)	99(63.9)
Pond/lake	3(1.9)	152(98.1)
Well	3(1.9)	152(98.1)
Spring	1(0.6)	154(99.4)
Sources of Water for Cooking		
Pipe water	65(43.2)	88(56.8)
Borehole	19(12.3)	136(87.7)
Rainwater	5(3.2)	150(96.8)
Dam	0(0.0)	155(100)
River water	55(35.5)	100(64.5)
Pond/lake	1(0.6)	154(99.4)
Well	1(0.6)	154(99.4)
Spring	0(0.0)	155(100)
Water treatment		
Boil	14(9.0)	141(91.0)
Add alum	15(9.7)	140(90.3)
Strain with Cloth	8(5.2)	147(94.8)

Characteristics	Total (n = 155), n (%)	Total (n = 155), n (%)
Filter	11(7.1)	144(92.9)
Sit and settle	36(23.2)	119(76.8)

Table 3.
Domestic attitudinal characteristics of study participants.

participants use pipe water as the major source of water for drinking, bathing, and cooking respectively. 23.2% of the participants treat their water by allowing it to sit and settle with only 9.7% and 9.0% of the participants stating that they use alum and boiling as a mode of water treatment respectively.

3.4 Practices in relation to schistosomiasis and soil-transmitted helminthic infections

Practices of study participants are presented in **Table 4**. 66.5% of the participants partake in farming. Also, 82.8%, 79.4%, and 16.3% of the participants wash their hands with water after visiting the toilet, wash their hands with both soap and water after visiting the toilet and wash their hands after playing on the ground respectively. More than half (62.6%) cross a river when going to the farm while 51.8% out of the 155 wear pairs of shoes when going to the farm.

3.5 Prevalence of schistosomiasis and other soil-transmitted helminths

The overall prevalence of helminthic infection among the school pupil after 21 days of mass drug administration was 11 (7.2%). There were only hookworm and *Schistosoma haematobium* treatment failure positives cases recorded after the MDA of the study participants. The study observed treatment failure of 3.3% and 3.9% for hookworm and *Schistosoma haematobium* infection respectively (**Table 5**).

3.6 Association between risk factors and helminthic infection

Helminthic infection was significantly associated with participants' source of drinking water (p = 0.013), number of individuals who share toilet facility (p = 0.049) and whether participants disposed garbage into a river (p = 0.015) (**Table 6**).

Characteristics	Total (n = 155), n (%)	Total (n = 155), n (%)
Practices/Behaviour	**Yes**	**No**
Do you partake in farming	103(66.5)	52(33.5)
Do you wear shoes when going to the farm	88(51.8)	67(43.2)
Do you cross a river when going	97(62.6)	58(37.4)
Do you wash your hands with water after visiting the toilet	128(82.8)	27(17.4)
Do you wash your hands with soap after visiting the toilet	123(79.4)	32(20.4)
Do you wash your hands after playing on the grounds	95(61.3)	60(38.7)
Do you come in contact with water bodies	129(83.2)	26(16.3)

Table 4.
Practices/behavioural characteristics of study participants (n = 155).

Categories	Positives (n = 153)	Prevalence (%)
Hookworm	5	3.3
Schistosoma haematobium	6	3.9
Overall Helminthic infections	11	7.2

Table 5.
Prevalence of helminthiasis after mass drug administration.

Variables	Helminth Positive n(%)	Helminth Negative n(%)	P-value
Source of drinking			
River			
Yes	8(13.8)	50(86.2)	**0.013**
No	3(7.2)	92(96.8)	
How many use toilet facility			
<5	1(4.2)	23(95.8)	**0.049**
>5	3(3.7)	79(96.3)	
Do not know	7(14.9)	40(85.1)	
Garbage disposal (River)			
Yes	2(20)	8(80)	**0.015**
No	8(5.7)	133(94.3)	
Do not know	1(50)	1(50)	

Associations between helminthic infection status and all other variables were assessed however, the only statistically significant association have been reported here.

Table 6.
Association between risk factors and helminth infection.

4. Discussion

Helminthic infection is very common among school children in Ghana. The Ministry of Health has been organising periodic MDA for school pupils. However, there have not been followed up exercises to assess the efficacy of the MDA among the school children in the Assin Manso community. Therefore, this study evaluates the effectiveness of the MDA and the knowledge, attitude and practice related to Schistosomiasis and STHs infection among the school pupils. This study revealed that most of the Basic School pupils have low knowledge (36.0%) about the modes of transmission of helminthic infections. This suggests that health education on helminthic infections as a control measure has not been effectively instituted particularly among pupils in the area, thus increasing their risk of acquiring helminthic infections. This observation is consistent with other findings in Bangladesh [13], Kenya [14], South Africa [15] and Ethiopia [16]. However, the finding contradicts the report by Sady, Al-Mekhlafi [17], who recorded higher awareness on the modes of transmissions among rural populations in Yemen. As highlighted in a study by Dawaki, Al-Mekhlafi [18], individuals living in remote rural neighbourhoods often lack the requisite knowledge on the causes, mode of transmission, signs, and symptoms, and preventive measures of schistosomiasis due to their poor economic status as reported by Murnane [19].

We found that the majority (70%) of the school children use untreated water for domestic purposes, which agrees with a report by Addo, Addo [20] in a Ghanaian community that 93% of the households do not treat their water before drinking. The continuous domestic use of untreated water is a risk factor for helminthic infections seeing that the river is the major source of water in the community. Unprotected surface water such as rivers, lakes, or springs or groundwater can easily become contaminated by human or animal faeces thus making the need for water treatment urgent [21].

The study also found that more than 60% of the participants engage in farming activities, with 62.6% reporting that they cross-river when going to their farms and 42.6% reporting that they do not wear shoes when going to the farm. This observation corroborates with the studies by Midzi, Mtapuri-Zinyowera [22], who reported that 82.6% of helminthiasis patients engage in farming. This could be an important risk factor for helminth infection since most of the farmers practise open range defecation and may shed some of the helminths eggs through their stools into the soil that could be picked up during farming practices thus increasing the risk of helminthic infections. Also, most of the farmers may come into body contact with water body sources that they cross to their various farms and these water bodies may be a major risk factor of schistosomiasis infection, since schistosomes present in the water bodies may penetrate the skin during surface body contact to cause the infections [23].

We observed that the majority (79.4%) of the children wash their hands with soap and water before eating, after visiting the toilet, and after playing on the grounds. This could be as a result of the promotion and enforcement of personal hygiene by school authorities, thus reducing the pupils' susceptibility to helminthic infections.

4.1 Association between risk factors and helminth infection

We found a significant association between the source of drinking water and helminthic infections which confirms the report by Tiruneh, Geshere [24], Adu-Gyasi, Asante [25], Simon-Oke, Afolabi [26], who identified the source of drinking water as a significant risk factor of helminthic infection. These studies revealed that the use of protected water sources such as pipe was associated with a reduced odds of helminthic infection [25], whereas the use of unprotected water sources such as rivers was associated with increased odds of infection [24]. Studies by Simon-Oke, Afolabi [26] also identified a high prevalence (45%) of helminthic infection among individuals whose major source of drinking water was the river and a relatively lower prevalence (10%) among pipe water users.

The study also observed a significant association between the sharing of toilet facilities and helminthic infections, which agrees with findings by Mahfouz, el-Morshedy [27], Heijnen, Cumming [28], who observed sharing of toilet facilities as a risk factor for helminthic infection. This could be attributed to the poor sanitary practices and the ease of disease spread which could be observed at shared toilet facilities, particularly communal toilet facilities.

Evidence from our study also indicates that poor garbage disposal practices such as the disposal of refuse into the river are associated with the contraction of helminthic infection. This was actually in line with studies by Curtale, Pezzotti [29], Asady, Ismail [30], who observed that improper garbage disposal was significantly associated with STH infection. This results from the fact that improper disposal of waste contaminated with helminth into soil often facilitates the spread of STH infection, particularly through the ingestion of eggs.

4.2 Treatment failure

We found a treatment failure rate of 7.2% among the school children who had received MDA less than a month ago. This indicates that some of the worms may have developed resistance to albendazole and praziquantel and this could pose a serious problem towards the eradication of these worms in the community. This finding is consistent with studies by Humphries, Mosites [31], Jaske [32], who both observed higher treatment failure of 39% and 36.8% respectively among individuals treated with albendazole. As highlighted by Humphries, Mosites [31], Humphries, Nguyen [33] this high rate of albendazole failure raises concern about emerging resistance particularly among STH endemic communities. A recent study done in the middle belt of Ghana found that comorbidity of STH with malaria parasites could increase albendazole treatment failure among individuals [34]. Thus we recommend if possible to screen the school children for malaria infection before MDA and possibly treating individuals with concurrent infection with both antimalaria and anthelminthic drugs. A recent study by Djune-Yemeli, Nana-Djeunga [35] also suggested that the use of Mebendazole- or Albendazole-based MDA alone among high-risk populations may not be sufficient to eliminate soil-transmitted helminthic infections thus necessitating the urgent need for new antihelminthics [36].

We found some treatment failure of praziquantel (PZQ) treatment against schistosomiasis infection among the school children and this is supportive of other studies findings of increased treatment failure of PZQ in certain communities in Ghana [37–43]. This finding is also supported by a systemic review and meta-analysis by Danso-Appiah and De Vlas [42], who provide corroborative evidence of the unexpectedly low cure rate associated with the use of praziquantel.

Whilst it is unclear the reason for the relatively high prevalence of treatment failures being recorded globally, particularly in endemic areas, various studies have suggested that factors underlying this observation include; the sub-curative efficacy of the typical dose of 40–60 mg/kg [44], the presence of immature worms and insufficient drug uptake particularly due to unique metabolic characteristics of specific patients [45] and helminths comorbidity with malaria [34].

5. Conclusion

This study revealed treatment failure of both albendazole and praziquantel against STH and Schistosomiasis infection, respectively among the Basic school children. Thus, we recommend mob up screening exercises after the MDA and treatment of children who may still test positive. This will contribute to the prevention and management of helminthic infections among school children. There is also the need to raise awareness about the issue of MDA failure to encourage all stakeholders to contribute towards control of helminthic infection through the development of better water purification systems to provide potable water and the provision of effective incinerators for proper waste disposal, to promote environmental hygiene... It is also necessary to improve health education, to enable pupils to avoid habits that lead to STH and schistosomiasis.

Author details

Benjamin Amoani[1*], Gideon Kwesi Nakotey[1], Samuel Asamoah Sakyi[2], Karen Pomeyie[1] and Christian Sewor[1]

1 Department of Biomedical Science, School of Allied Health Sciences, University of Cape Coast, Cape Coast, Ghana

2 Molecular Medicine Department, School of Medical Sciences, Kwame Nkrumah University of Science and Technology, Ghana

*Address all correspondence to: bamoani@ucc.edu.gh

References

[1] Munisi DZ, Buza J, Mpolya EA, Angelo T, Kinung'hi SM. Knowledge, attitude, and practices on intestinal schistosomiasis among primary schoolchildren in the Lake Victoria basin, Rorya District, North-Western Tanzania. BMC Public Health. 2017;**17**(1):731. DOI: 10.1186/s12889-017-4767-9

[2] Sacolo H, Chimbari M, Kalinda C. Knowledge, attitudes and practices on schistosomiasis in sub-Saharan Africa: A systematic review. BMC Infectious Diseases. 2018;**18**(1):46. DOI: 10.1186/s12879-017-2923-6

[3] WHO. Foodborne Disease Outbreaks: Guidelines for Investigation and Control. Geneva: World Health Organization; 2008

[4] Brooker S, Kabatereine NB, Smith JL, Mupfasoni D, Mwanje MT, Ndayishimiye O, et al. An updated atlas of human helminth infections: The example of East Africa. International Journal of Health Geographics. 2009;**8**(1):42. DOI: 10.1186/1476-072X-8-42

[5] Ahiadorme M, Morhe E. Soil transmitted helminth infections in Ghana: A ten year review. The Pan African Medical Journal. 2020;**35**:131. DOI: 10.11604/pamj.2020.35.131.21069

[6] Mirisho R, Neizer ML, Sarfo B. Prevalence of intestinal Helminths infestation in children attending Princess Marie Louise Children's Hospital in Accra, Ghana. Journal of Parasitology Research. 2017;**2017**:8524985. DOI: 10.1155/2017/8524985

[7] WHO. Preventive Chemotherapy in Human Helminthiasis. Coordinated Use of Anthelminthic Drugs in Control Interventions: A Manual for Health Professionals and Programme Managers. Geneva: World Health Organization; 2006

[8] Awasthi S, Bundy DA, Savioli L. Helminthic infections. BMJ. 2003;**327**(7412):431-433. DOI: 10.1136/bmj.327.7412.431

[9] Sowemimo OA, Asaolu SO. Current status of soil-transmitted helminthiases among pre-school and school-aged children from Ile-Ife, Osun state, Nigeria. Journal of Helminthology. 2011;**85**(3):234-238. DOI: 10.1017/S0022149X10000489

[10] Rassi C, Kajungu D, Martin S, Arroz J, Tallant J, Zegers de Beyl C, et al. Have you heard of schistosomiasis? Knowledge, attitudes and practices in Nampula Province, Mozambique. PLoS Neglected Tropical Diseases. 2016;**10**(3):e0004504. DOI: 10.1371/journal.pntd.0004504

[11] USAID. END in Africa: USAID; 2015. Available from: http://endinafrica.org/challenge/program-challenges/

[12] The Partnership for Child Development. The cost of large-scale school health programmes which deliver anthelmintics to children in Ghana and Tanzania. Acta Tropica. 1999;**73**(2):183-204. DOI: 10.1016/s0001-706x(99)00028-5

[13] Nath TC, Padmawati RS, Alam MS, Das S, Murhandarwati EH. Elimination of soil-transmitted helminthiasis infection in Bangladesh: knowledge, attitudes, and practices regarding mass drug administration. Journal of Global Health Reports. 1 Jun 2018:e2018017. DOI: 10.29392/joghr.2.e2018017

[14] Masaku J, Mutungi F, Gichuki PM, Okoyo C, Njomo DW, Njenga SM. High prevalence of helminths infection and associated risk factors among adults living in a rural setting, Central Kenya: A cross-sectional study. Tropical Medicine and Health. 2017;**45**(1):15. DOI: 10.1186/s41182-017-0055-8

[15] Sibiya JE, Gumbo JR. Knowledge, attitude and practices (KAP) survey on water, sanitation and hygiene in selected schools in Vhembe District, Limpopo, South Africa. International Journal of Environmental Research and Public Health. 2013;**10**(6):2282-2295. DOI: 10.3390/ijerph10062282

[16] Vivas AP, Gelaye B, Aboset N, Kumie A, Berhane Y, Williams MA. Knowledge, attitudes and practices (KAP) of hygiene among school children in Angolela, Ethiopia. Journal of Preventive Medicine and Hygiene. 2010;**51**(2):73-79

[17] Sady H, Al-Mekhlafi HM, Atroosh WM, Al-Delaimy AK, Nasr NA, Dawaki S, et al. Knowledge, attitude, and practices towards schistosomiasis among rural population in Yemen. Parasites & Vectors. 2015;**8**(1):436. DOI: 10.1186/s13071-015-1050-8

[18] Dawaki S, Al-Mekhlafi HM, Ithoi I, Ibrahim J, Abdulsalam AM, Ahmed A, et al. Prevalence and Risk Factors of Schistosomiasis among Hausa Communities in Kano State, Nigeria. Revista do Instituto de Medicina Tropical de São Paulo. 2016;**58**:54. DOI: 10.1590/S1678-9946201658054

[19] Murnane RJ. Improving the education of children living in poverty. The Future of Children. 2007;**17**(2):161-182. DOI: 10.1353/foc.2007.0019

[20] Addo HO, Addo KK, LangBong B. Water handling and hygiene practices on the transmission of diarrhoeal diseases and soil transmitted helminthic infections in communities in rural Ghana. Civil and Environmental Research. 2014;**6**(1):68-79

[21] Vaz Nery S, Pickering AJ, Abate E, Asmare A, Barrett L, Benjamin-Chung J, et al. The role of water, sanitation and hygiene interventions in reducing soil-transmitted helminths: interpreting the evidence and identifying next steps. Parasit Vectors. 2019;**12**(1):273. DOI: 10.1186/s13071-019-3532-

[22] Midzi N, Mtapuri-Zinyowera S, Mapingure MP, Paul NH, Sangweme D, Hlerema G, et al. Knowledge attitudes and practices of grade three primary schoolchildren in relation to schistosomiasis, soil transmitted helminthiasis and malaria in Zimbabwe. BMC Infectious Diseases. 2011;**11**:169. DOI: 10.1186/1471-2334-11-169

[23] Wakelin D. Helminths: Pathogenesis and Defenses. In: Baron S, editors. Medical Microbiology. Galveston (TX): University of Texas Medical Branch at Galveston

[24] Tiruneh T, Geshere G, Ketema T. Prevalence and determinants of soil-transmitted helminthic infections among school children at Goro primary school, south west Shewa, Ethiopia. International Journal of Pediatrics. 2020;**2020**:8612054. DOI: 10.1155/2020/8612054

[25] Adu-Gyasi D, Asante KP, Frempong MT, Gyasi DK, Iddrisu LF, Ankrah L, et al. Epidemiology of soil transmitted helminth infections in the middle-belt of Ghana, Africa. Parasite Epidemiology and Control. 2018;**3**(3):e00071. DOI: 10.1016/j.parepi.2018.e00071

[26] Simon-Oke IA, Afolabi OJ, Obimakinde ET. Parasitic contamination

of water sources in Akure, Ondo state, Nigeria. The Journal of Basic and Applied Zoology. 2020;**81**(1):50. DOI: 10.1186/s41936-020-00187-7

[27] Mahfouz AA, el-Morshedy H, Farghaly A, Khalil A. Ecological determinants of intestinal parasitic infections among pre-school children in an urban squatter settlement of Egypt. Journal of Tropical Pediatrics. 1997;**43**(6):341-344. DOI: 10.1093/tropej/43.6.341

[28] Heijnen M, Cumming O, Peletz R, Chan GK, Brown J, Baker K, et al. Shared sanitation versus individual household latrines: A systematic review of health outcomes. PLoS One. 2014;**9**(4):e93300. DOI: 10.1371/journal.pone.0093300

[29] Curtale F, Pezzotti P, Saad YS, Aloi A. An analysis of individual, household, and environmental risk factors for intestinal helminth infection among children in Qena governorate, Upper Egypt. Journal of Tropical Pediatrics. 1999;**45**(1):14-17. DOI: 10.1093/tropej/45.1.14

[30] Asady A, Ismail S, Abdul Jalil M, Pakeer O. Soil Transmitted Helminth Infection among Children Admitted to Hospital Tengku Ampuan Afzan, Kuantan, Pahang. IIUM Medical Journal Malaysia. 2019;**18**(2):107. DOI: 10.31436/imjm.v18i2.89

[31] Humphries D, Mosites E, Otchere J, Twum WA, Woo L, Jones-Sanpei H, et al. Epidemiology of hookworm infection in Kintampo north municipality, Ghana: Patterns of malaria coinfection, anemia, and albendazole treatment failure. The American Journal of Tropical Medicine and Hygiene. 2011;**84**(5):792-800. DOI: 10.4269/ajtmh.2011.11-0003

[32] Jaske E. An Assessment of Hookworm Infection and Albendazole Treatment Failure among Children Ages 7-12 In Kintampo North Municipality, Ghana. New Haven, Connecticut: Yale University; 2014

[33] Humphries D, Nguyen S, Boakye D, Wilson M, Cappello M. The promise and pitfalls of mass drug administration to control intestinal helminth infections. Current Opinion in Infectious Diseases. 2012;**25**(5):584-589. DOI: 10.1097/QCO.0b013e328357e4cf

[34] Amoani B, Adu B, Frempong M, Barnes P, Cappello M, Gyan B, et al. Necator americanus and plasmodium falciparum co-infection and albendazole treatment outcome among individuals in rural Ghana. The Journal of Advances in Parasitology. 2019;**6**(4):51-54

[35] Djune-Yemeli L, Nana-Djeunga HC, Lenou-Nanga CG, Donfo-Azafack C, Domche A, Fossuo-Thotchum F, et al. Serious limitations of the current strategy to control soil-transmitted Helminths and added value of Ivermectin/Albendazole mass administration: A population-based observational study in Cameroon. PLoS Neglected Tropical Diseases. 2020;**14**(11):e0008794. DOI: 10.1371/journal.pntd.0008794

[36] Keiser J, Utzinger J. Efficacy of current drugs against soil-transmitted helminth infections: Systematic review and meta-analysis. Journal of the American Medical Association. 2008;**299**(16):1937-1948. DOI: 10.1001/jama.299.16.1937

[37] Alonso D, Munoz J, Gascon J, Valls ME, Corachan M. Failure of standard treatment with praziquantel in two returned travelers with Schistosoma haematobium infection. The American Journal of Tropical Medicine and Hygiene. 2006;**74**(2):342-344

[38] Utzinger J, N'Goran EK, N'Dri A, Lengeler C, Tanner M. Efficacy of praziquantel against Schistosoma mansoni with particular consideration for intensity of infection. Tropical Medicine &

International Health. 2000;**5**(11):771-778. DOI: 10.1046/j.1365-3156.2000.00646.x

[39] Midzi N, Sangweme D, Zinyowera S, Mapingure MP, Brouwer KC, Kumar N, et al. Efficacy and side effects of praziquantel treatment against Schistosoma haematobium infection among primary school children in Zimbabwe. Transactions of the Royal Society of Tropical Medicine and Hygiene. 2008;**102**(8):759-766. DOI: 10.1016/j.trstmh.2008.03.010

[40] Silva IM, Pereira Filho E, Thiengo R, Ribeiro PC, Conceicao MJ, Panasco M, et al. Schistosomiasis haematobia: Histopathological course determined by cystoscopy in a patient in whom praziquantel treatment failed. Revista do Instituto de Medicina Tropical de São Paulo. 2008;**50**(6):343-346. DOI: 10.1590/s0036-46652008000600006

[41] Silva IM, Thiengo R, Conceicao MJ, Rey L, Lenzi HL, Pereira Filho E, et al. Therapeutic failure of praziquantel in the treatment of Schistosoma haematobium infection in Brazilians returning from Africa. Memórias do Instituto Oswaldo Cruz. 2005;**100**(4):445-449. DOI: 10.1590/s0074-02762005000400018

[42] Danso-Appiah A, De Vlas SJ. Interpreting low praziquantel cure rates of Schistosoma mansoni infections in Senegal. Trends in Parasitology. 2002;**18**(3):125-129. DOI: 10.1016/s1471-4922(01)02209-7

[43] Lawn SD, Lucas SB, Chiodini PL. Case report: Schistosoma mansoni infection: Failure of standard treatment with praziquantel in a returned traveller. Transactions of the Royal Society of Tropical Medicine and Hygiene. 2003;**97**(1):100-101. DOI: 10.1016/s0035-9203(03)90038-1

[44] Doenhoff MJ, Pica-Mattoccia L. Praziquantel for the treatment of schistosomiasis: Its use for control in areas with endemic disease and prospects for drug resistance. Expert Review of Anti-Infective Therapy. 2006;**4**(2): 199-210. DOI: 10.1586/14787210.4.2.199

[45] Botros S, Sayed H, Amer N, El-Ghannam M, Bennett JL, Day TA. Current status of sensitivity to praziquantel in a focus of potential drug resistance in Egypt. International Journal for Parasitology. 2005;**35**(7):787-791. DOI: 10.1016/j.ijpara.2005.02.005

Chapter 5

One Health Concept against Schistosomiasis: An Overview

Tonay Inceboz

Abstract

Schistosomiasis (bilharziasis) is a parasitic disease caused by *Schistosoma* spp. that belongs to trematode worms. These worms are known as "blood parasites". This disease is included in "neglected tropical diseases" and "water-borne diseases". The main species are *Schistosoma* (S.) *haematobium, S. japonicum, S. mansoni, S. intercalatum, S. mekongi, S. guineensis* and *S. intercalatum*, though there are more than 20 different species. The parasite in the definitive host may affect many organs and systems. The disease may become chronic and lasts 3–8 years and even up to 20–30 years. The definitive host is primarily human; however, in endemic areas animals such as monkeys, cattle, horses, rodents, cats, dogs are reservoirs. According to World Health Organization (WHO), schistosomiasis affects 250 million people, and causes 1.9 million deaths yearly in endemic areas. Moreover, due to global warming, the spread of the disease may increase. The effective way to fight against schistosomiasis is following the "one-health system". Indeed, to overcome or "eradicate" this disease, we have to strive against different forms at different evolutionary stages of the worm such as, forms in humans, domestic or wild animals, and freshwater snails. If we combine the knowledge of professionals, we may achieve this goal.

Keywords: *schistosoma* spp., schistosomiasis, epidemiology, one health concept

1. Introduction

Schistosoma spp. spread over many continents around the world, primarily in Asia, Africa, and America. There are more than 20 types of *Schistosoma* in the world. This speciation is most likely due to differences in intermediate hosts and definitive hosts [1–3].

The 250 million cases of Schistosomiasis reported globally by WHO are distributed among different countries as follows:

In Africa; Nigeria 26.21%, Ethiopia 9.57%, the Democratic Republic of the Congo 7.74%, Mozambique 5.82%, Kenya 5.04%, United Republic of Tanzania 4.32%, Cameroon 4.30%, Uganda 3.66%, Malawi 2.89%, and Ghana 2.88%. Furthermore, there are high-risk countries such as Angola, Benin, Botswana, Burkina

IntechOpen

Faso, Burundi, Central African Republic, Chad, Côte d'Ivoire, Equatorial Guinea, Eritrea, Gabon, Gambia, Guinea, Guinea-Bissau, Liberia, Madagascar, Malawi, Mali, Mauritania, Namibia, Niger, Rwanda, São Tomé and Príncipe, Senegal, Sierra Leone, Republic of South Africa, Eswatini, Togo, Uganda, Zambia, and Zimbabwe [4]. Although they are located in the African continent; Morocco, Tunisia, and Algeria are at low risk for schistosomiasis [3, 5, 6].

Of the schistosomiasis cases in the Americas, 95.80% are in Brazil and 4.20% in the Bolivarian Republic of Venezuela [4]. *Schistosoma mansoni* is the only species present in Latin American and Caribbean countries [3]. It has been estimated that around 25 million people are at risk in the Americas. The risk is a "big public health problem," especially in freshwater lakes and rivers in Southeastern Brazil, whereas St. Lucia and Suriname are at lower risk [7, 8].

In the Eastern Mediterranean region, the prevalence of schistosomiasis is 57.85% in Yemen, 38.36% in Sudan, 3.39% in Somalia, and 0.40% in Egypt. Iraq, Libya, Oman, Saudi Arabia, and Syrian Arab Republic are low-risk countries for Schistosomiasis. In the Western Pacific region, the Philippines (78.28%), China (19.37%), Lao People's Democratic Republic (1.41%), and Cambodia (0.94%) are reported as endemic countries. Indonesia is an endemic country in South-East Asia, whereas India and Thailand have low risk. There have not been any reported cases in the European continent (**Figure 1**) [4].

The first tussle against schistosomiasis was via intravenous tartar emetic, a derivative of antimony, in Egypt and Sudan in 1920 [10]. Recently, WHO released a strategic plan under sustainable development objectives, aiming for the "total eradication of schistosomiasis," which is an important public health target for the affected 78 countries and others [4, 11]. "Total eradication" is defined as the reduction of serious forms of schistosomiasis down to <1% [12]. According to WHO's plan (intestinal treat all school-age children, also treat adults considered to be at and urogenital schistosomiasis), praziquantel treatment is expected to decrease morbidity as well as eradicate the disease. Additional protection measures such as, preventing water contamination and increasing awareness through education are the other tools to combat the disease (**Figure 2**) [11].

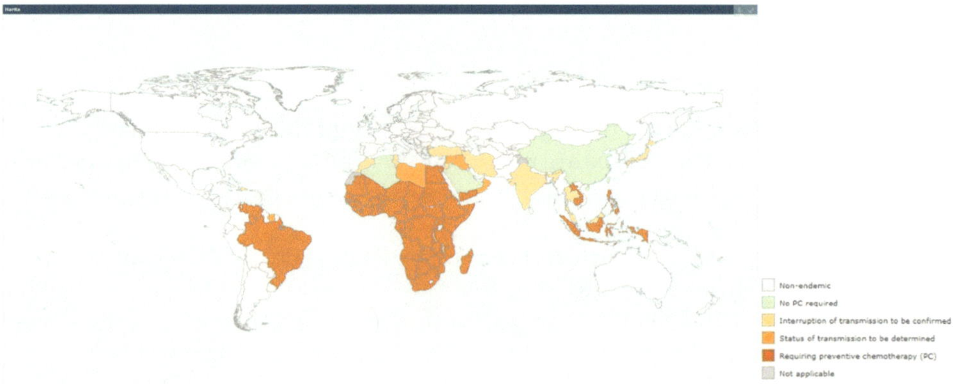

Figure 1.
This map shows the distribution of schistosomiasis in the world [9]. Link: https://apps.who.int/neglected_diseases/ntddata/sch/sch.html

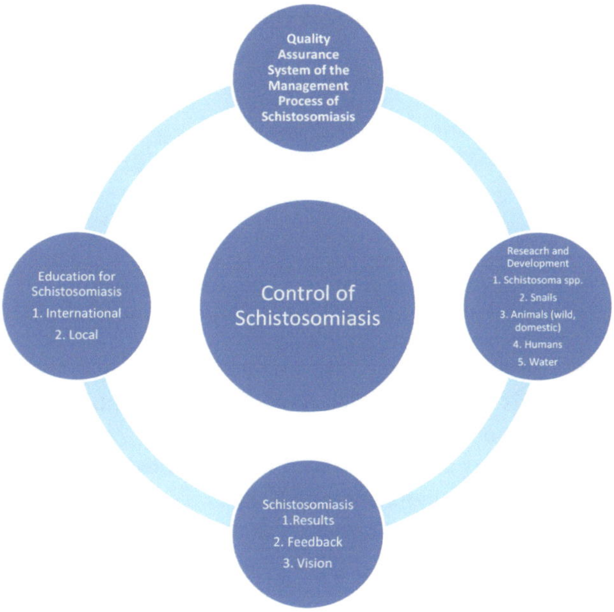

Figure 2.
Control of schistosomiasis.

2. Quality assurance system of the management process of schistosomiasis

2.1 International organizations

There are many programs and organizations that work towards finding solutions against schistosomiasis such as WHO disability-adjusted life years (DALY), World Health Assembly (WHA), neglected tropical diseases (NTDs), soil-transmitted helminthiases (STH), and waterborne diseases [11]. Defining prudential targets according to previous data:

2.2 Local organizations

Local organizations have pivotal roles in combatting schistosomiasis. In Brazil, for instance, there are many organizations fighting against the disease: Schistosomiasis Control Programme (PCE), Secretary of Public Health Surveillance (SVS), the Secretary of Health in the State of Minas Gerais (SESMG), Superintendência de Controle de Endemias, Instituto Nacional de Pesquisas Espaciais, Centro de Pesquisas René Rachou. There are also some environmental institutes in Brazil such as moderate resolution imaging spectroradiometer (MODIS), the shuttle radar topography mission (SRTM), Center for Weather Forecast and Climate Studies (CPTEC) [11]. This "fight" should be handled in coordination with the Ministries of Health, Education, Agriculture, and Environment in endemic regions. This would be the most logical solution against parasitic infections because of the different life-cycle periods in intermediate/definitive hosts of the parasites.

I guess there is a Bilharziasis Institute in Egypt.

3. The field of Research and Development

3.1 *Schistosoma* species

life cycle, diagnosis, epidemiology, geographic distribution, treatment, prevention, vaccines, etc.

3.2 Animals

3.2.1 Snails

Considering the "One Health Concept," one of the most important elements to combat schistosomiasis is to prevent ecologic and geographic dissemination of *Schistosoma* during the development of snails [13, 14].

Infected definitive hosts, namely humans and the above-mentioned animals release *Schistosoma* eggs. When eggs become in contact with aquatic environment, miracidia – the second form of *Schistosoma* – develops in the eggs. Then, miracidia penetrate the snails and become still-sporocysts. These sporocysts transform into motile baby sporocysts by internal budding. This is followed by migration of baby sporocysts to the digestive system of the snails, where the sporocysts grow all their glands through cylinder-like processes. Many cercariae develop from tubules of sporocysts. Cercariae are freed from snails via rupture of the tubules. This process, from miracidium to cercaria, takes around 3–12 weeks [15].

Intermediate hosts for *Schistosoma mansoni*, *Schistosoma haematobium,* and *S. japonicum* are the snails *Biomphalaria glabrata, Bulinus* spp., and *Oncomelania hupensis* ssp., respectively. In Brazil, however, intermediate hosts for *S. mansoni* also include *Biomphalaria tenagophila* (Orbigny, 1835), *Basilodes straminea (*Dunker, 1848) *B. peregrina* (Orbigny, 1835), *B. schrammi* (Crosse, 1864), *B. kuhniana* (Clessin, 1883), *B. intermedia* (Paraense & Deslandes, 1962), *B. amazonica* (Paraense, 1966), *B. oligoza*

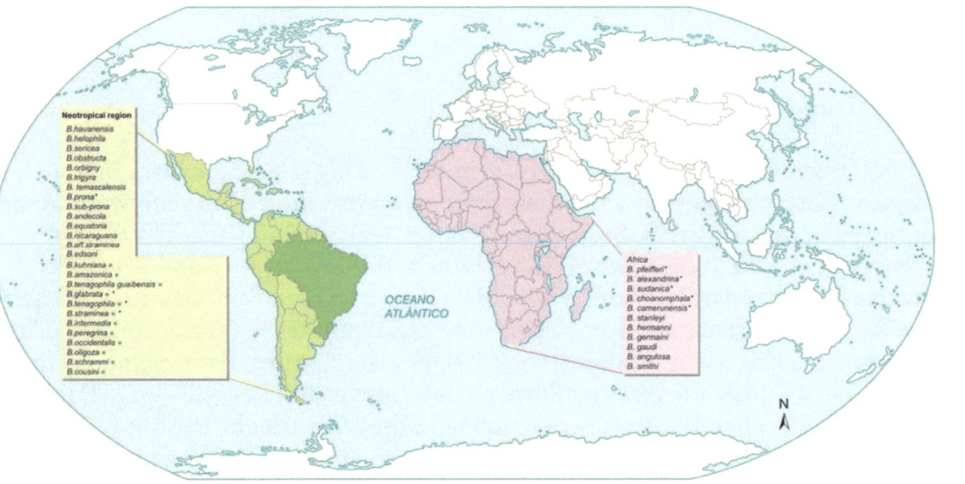

Figure 3.
This map shows the distribution of Biomphalaria species in the World (according Palasio, R.G.S., 2011) [17, 18]. Link: https://www.academia.edu/17716515/Pattern_of_Genetic_Divergence_of_Mitochondrial_DNA_Sequences_in_Biomphalaria_tenagophila_Complex_Species_Based_on_Barcode_and_Morphological_Analysis

(Paraense, 1974), *B. occidentalis* (Paraense, 1981), *B. cousini* (Paraense, 1966), and *B. tenagophila guaibensis* (Paraense, 1984).

The map (Figure XX) below demonstrates the worldwide distribution of the thirty-seven *Biomphalaria* species, the twenty-six neotropical *Biomphalaria* species, and the eleven snail species, and one subspecies naturally described in Brazil. An asterisk indicates *S. mansoni* host species [16–18].

To identify the *Schistosoma* from snails, many molecular-based techniques such as PCR, qPCR, loop-mediated isothermal amplification (LAMP), environmental DNA analysis (eDNA), and droplet digital PCR (ddPCR) are commonly used [15].

The relationship of snail species (intermediate host) with *Schistosoma* spp. as well as with predator fish should be investigated. This would be a good area for future research. It is also essential to preserve the ecological balance and prevent anthropogenic harm to nature (**Figure 3**).

3.2.2 Domestic animals

It is of utmost importance to look for faunas of infection in wild and farm animals as definitive hosts and snails as intermediate hosts. Definitive hosts for *Schistosoma* spp. in animals are: *S. bovis* in cattle; *S. mattheei* in sheep and goats; *Cercopithecus sabaus* in monkeys; *S. indicum*, *S. spindale,* and *S.nasale* in horses, swines, and dogs; and *S. japonicum* in dogs [19].

3.2.3 Wild animals

In which region, where wild animals may be infected by *Schistosoma* spp. should be considered.

In Brazil, there are shrewmice (*Oxymycterus sp.*, *Necromys lasiurus*, *Holochilus spp.*, *Akodon spp.*, *Sooretamys spp.*, *Calomys spp.*, *Proechimys sp.*, *Cavia aperea*, and *Rattus rattus* and *Rattus norvegicus*) infected with *Schistosoma* spp. (*S. manoni*, *S. bovis*, *Sirthenea rodhaini* ve *S. kisumuensis*). *S. malayensis* can be found in Mueller mice (*Rattus muelleri*) in Malaysia; however, it is rare to be present in humans. *S. ovuncatum* and *S. sinesium* were found in *R. rattus* in Thailand [20, 21].

The research in Senegal revealed that there was hybridization between *S. bovis* and *S. haematobium*, between *S. haematobium* and *S. curassoni* in humans, and between *S. bovis* and *S. curassoni* in cattle [22, 23].

3.2.4 Humans

It is important to know which *Schistosoma* spp. may cause infection in humans in different regions, and how human organs would respond in reaction to such infections.

If snails are infected with *Schistosoma* spp. cercariae can be released into the freshwater bodies such as lakes and rivers. Humans may become infected if these cercariae perforate and enter through the skin. This may cause inflammation, papule formation, and itching on the skin. In addition, if humans drink the infected water that contains cercariae, the infection may occur via the mucosal route [4].

Schistosoma spp. infection may cause the involvement of many organs and systems in human, such as the liver, lungs, heart, gastrointestinal tractus, and urogenital system.

There are two phases of the *Schistosoma* infection in humans. In the acute phase, common symptoms are fever, cough, rash, arthralgia, malaise, anorexia, vomiting, and diarrhea [1]. “Katayama syndrome” is one of the early clinical effects in hypersensitive patients infected with *Schistosoma* spp. (*Schistosoma mansoni*, *S. japonicum*). It occurs within 14–84 days of infection and is manifested by nocturnal fever, cough, myalgia, headache, and abdominal tenderness [1, 24, 25].

In the chronic phase of schistosomiasis, clinical findings such as vaginal bleeding, dysuria, hematuria, anemia, bladder carcinoma (*S. haematobium*), hematochezia, cirrhosis, neurological problems, and even death may occur [1, 24].

Schistosomiasis is a treatable disease if diagnosed. Thus, awareness of this disease and early diagnosis is very important to eradicate it.

3.2.5 Water

Stream, river, lake, pond, waterfall, fluvial environment, flora, flood, dams, and drainage systems are key elements in the spread of *Schistosoma* spp.

Many problems are arising due to global warming, one of which is heavier flooding [26]. Floodwater may lead to exposure of humans and animals to infected water, mainly in endemic areas. Especially, *S. mansoni, S. japonicum, S. haematobium, S. mekongi, S. intercalatum*, and *S. guineensis* are considered waterborne parasites [27]. As a result of floods, flood fighters, as well as the public, may be at risk of infection [28, 29]. In addition, more than 40 different animal species may become infected by consuming contaminated water. These animals are not only farm animals such as cattle and sheep but also wild animals such as mice, rats, and deer in the nature [30–32]. One should be cautious when grassing the farm animals immediately after the flood. It is also necessary to detect and isolate the infected animals. There is unfortunately no preventive measure of control for *Schistosoma* in wild animals except sampling and examining.

The countries especially located in endemic areas should consider their ecological circumstances and receive consultation before building dams. Early warning systems for floods should be developed. Infectivity and potential risks of snail habitats should be evaluated in areas surrounding dams. The preventive measures against allowing the snails in drinking water and farming water springs should be taken. In the case of presence of infected snails in dam-water, the use of molluscicides should be considered [30, 33–35].

4. Education

4.1 Training of educators

Multidisciplinary international meetings should be held to define strategies for action plans against schistosomiasis.

4.2 Public education

People at risk – especially in endemic areas – such as young groups, soldiers, security forces, foresters, government officers, mountaineers, and water sporters should be trained periodically.

Species	**Natural definitive host species (excluding humans)**	**Human public health importance**	**intermediate host snail**	**Molluscivores**	**Geographic Distribution**	**References**
1. Mansoni group						
1.1.Schistosoma mansoni	Nonhuman primates (including apes), rodents, insectivores, artiodactylids (waterbuck), procyonids (raccoon)	High	*Biomphalaria pfeifferi*		Africa, Middle East, South America, (Brazil, Venezuela,Surinam) Caribbean	[36]
1.2. Schistosoma edwardiense	Hippopotamus		*Biomphalaria sudanica, Bulinus truncatus, or Ceratophallus natalensis.*		Lake Edward, Western Uganda	[37]
1.3.Schistosoma hippopotami	Wild, hippopotamus Artiodactyilds		*Biomphalaria sudanica, Bulinus truncatus, or Ceratophallus natalensis.*		Africa	[37]
1.4.Schistosoma rodhaini	Wild rodents, never in human beings.		*Planorbis* (*P. pfeifferi*), *P. tanganikanus*, African (*P. boissyi = P. alexandrina*), American (*P. glabratus*)		Africa, Congo Elisabethville, Albertville and Sakania,	[37]
2.Haematobium group						
2.1.Schistosoma haematobium	Humans, Nonhuman primates (not apes), artiodactylids (pigs, buffalo)	High	*Bulinus globosus* *Bulinusnyassanus* *B. truncatus* *B. succinoides*	*Trematocranus placodon*	Africa, Middle East	[38]
2.2.Schistosoma intercalatum	Humans, Possibly rodents	Low	*Bulinus* spp		Central Africa (D.R. Congo only)	[39]
2.3.Schistosoma bovis	Wild Artiodactyla, domestic (cattle, goats, sheep, horses and camels) artiodactyls	Low	*Bulinus* spp. *B. globosus*, *Beroe forskalii*, *Baebius nyassanus* and *B. truncatus*), *Planorbarius metidjensis*		in Africa north of the equator, Europe (Sardinia, Corsica, Spain), and the Middle East as far as Iraq	[40, 41]

Species	Natural definitive host species (excluding humans)	Human public health importance	intermediate host snail	Molluscivores	Geographic Distribution	References
2.4.Schistosoma curassoni	domestic artiodactyls(cattle, sheep, and goats)	Low			Africa	[22]
2.5.Schistosoma guineensis	Humans, Possibly rodents	Low	*Bulinus forskalii*		West Africa (Lower Guinea)	[42]
2.6.Schistosoma kisumuensis	Rodents, non-human primates, Artiodactyls		*Bulinus*		Africa, Lake Victoria Basin, Kenya	[20, 21]
2.7.Schistosoma leiperi	Wild artiodactyls, (antelope), BALB/c mice and in *Mastomys coucha* domestic artiodactyls	Low	*Bulinus*		Africa	[43]
2.8.Schistosoma margrebowiei	Wild artiodactyls (antelope), BALB/c mice, and in *M. coucha*, domestic artiodactyls	Low	*Bulinus natalensis*		Africa	[43]
2.9.Schistosoma mattheei	Humans, Nonhuman primates (not apes), Wild artiodactyls (cattle, antelope), domestic artiodactyls	Low	*Bulinus globosus*		Southern Africa	[44]
3.Indicum group						
3.1.Schistosoma indicum (pulmonary Schistosomiasis)	Domestic artiodactyls, (sheep, goat, water buffalo, cattle, camel, horse, donkey, dog, but not pigs) perissodactyls		*Indoplanorbis exustus*, *Lymnaea luteola*		W&S Asia, India and other Asian countries	[45–47]
3.2.Schistosoma nasale (nasal cavity)	domestic artiodactyls, buffaloes		*Bithynia tentaculata*, *Indoplanorbis exustus*		W&S Asia	[19]

Species	Natural definitive host species (excluding humans)	Human public health importance	intermediate host snail	Molluscivores	Geographic Distribution	References
3.3.Schistosoma spindale (examining mesentery of the animals)	Humans (dermatit), domestic artiodactyls (cattle, *water buffaloes (Bubalus bubalis),* goats (Artiodactyla, Ruminantia, *Bandicota indica, Rattus argentivente, Rattus diardi, Rattus tiomanicus jalorensis*		*Indoplanorbis exustus*		W&S Asia Bangladesh, South India, Malaysia	[48, 49]
4.Japonicum group						
4.1.Schistosoma japonicum	Humans, Nonhuman primates, artiodactylids (cats, dogs, goats, horses, pigs, water buffalos in particular), carnivores, rodents, perissodactylids (horses)	High	*Oncomelania hupensis*		East Asia (China, Philippines, Indonesia)	[50]
4.2.Schistosoma malayensis	Humans, Rodents (van Mueller's rat) *Sundamys muelleri*	Low	*Robertsiella* (*R. gismanni*, *R. kaporensis* și, *R. silvicola*		Southeast Asia Peninsular Malaysia	[20, 21]
4.3.Schistosoma mekongi	Humans, domestic artiodactyls, carnivors (dogs), Carnivoresartiodactylids(pigs)	Moderate	*Tricula aperta*		SE Asia (Vietnam, Cambodia, Laos, Thailand)	[24, 51]
4.4.Schistosoma ovuncatum	Rodents, nonhuman primates *Rattus rattus*, Laboratory host: *Mus musculus*		*Tricula bollingi*		Thailand and Southeast Asian	[52]
4.5.Schistosoma sinensium	Rodents, and laboratory rabbits		*Tricula bollingi* *Tricula* (pomatiopsida:*Triculinae)* *T. hortensis*		E&SE Asia Southern China, southeast Asia, and Northern India	[53, 54]
Schistosoma incognitum	Pigs, dogs and a variety of rodents (*R. Rattus*)		*Radix rubiginosa*		Asia southeastern India (Bengal), Java, and Thailand	[55]

Species	Natural definitive host species (excluding humans)	Human public health importance	intermediate host snail	Molluscivores	Geographic Distribution	References
5. New species (Orientobilharzia differs)						
5.1.*Schistosoma turkestanicum*	Cattle, sheep, goats, buffaloes	portal veins or intestinal veins	*Radix luteola*		Asia, China, India, Mongolia, Pakistan, Iraq, and Iran in Asia, and Russia	[47]
5.2.*Schistosoma bomfordi*			*Lymnaea rubiginosa, Radix luteola*		Nepal	[47]
5.3.*Schistosoma datta*						
5.4.*Schistosoma harinasutai*	Buffaloe		*Radix rubiginosa*		Thailand, Southern Laos	[56]
6. Hybrids						
6.1.*S. haematobium-S. guineenis* hybris (1996)					Cameroon	[57]
6.2. *S. mansoni-Sirthenea rodhaini* hybrid (2003)					Kenya	[58]
6.3. *S. haematobium–S. bovis* hybrids (2009)					Senegalese, Corsica	[22, 59]
6.4. *S. haematobium–S. mansoni* hybrid (2019)					Côte d'Ivoire.	[60]

Table 1.
Schematic phylogeny of interrelationships between members of the genus Schistosoma and definitive host and intermediate host vertebrates.

WHO's course of action set out the targets as eradicating schistosomiasis until 2025 (**Table 1**) [61].

5. Conclusion

1. Schistosomiasis is a "neglected disease" around the world.

2. Schistosomiasis is a waterborne disease.

3. *Schistosoma* spp. is present in humans and animals, which are definitive hosts in both urban and rural areas.

4. There is a risk of an increase in schistosomiasis due to global warming in tropical and subtropical areas.

5. Bioturbation due to dams, factories, and drainage systems should be avoided since these may cause an increase in *Schistosoma spp.* and further differentiation of *Schistosoma* spp. into new types.

6. If necessary, double-layer gloves and waterproof boots should be used in contact with infected water. If there is a direct skin contact, alcohol swabs should be used. Drinking water should be boiled and vegetables should be cooked before consumption, particularly in endemic areas [35].

Considering the "One Health Concept," all related individuals and groups, including parasitologists, veterinarians, public health professionals, biologists, molecular biologists, and geographers should work hand-in-hand to prevent, detect, treat, and eradicate Schistosomiasis.

Author details

Tonay Inceboz
Dokuz Eylül University, Turkey

*Address all correspondence to: tonay.inceboz@gmail.com

References

[1] Meltzer E, Schwartz E. Schistosomiasis: Current epidemiology and management in travelers. Current Infectious Disease Reports. 2013;**15**:211-215. DOI: 10.1007/s11908-013-0329-1

[2] Zoni AC, Catalá L, Ault SK. Schistosomiasis prevalence and intensity of infection in Latin America and the Caribbean countries, 1942-2014: A systematic review in the context of a regional elimination goal. PLoS Neglected Tropical Diseases. 2016;**10**:e0004493. DOI: 10.1371/journal.pntd.0004493

[3] Colley DG, Bustinduy AL, Secor WE, King CH. Human schistosomiasis. Lancet. 2014;**383**:2253-2264. DOI: 10.1016/S0140-6736(13)61949-2

[4] World Health Organization. Schistosomiasis (Bilharzia). Available from: https://www.who.int/health-topics/schistosomiasis#tab=tab_1 [Accessed: June 6, 2022]

[5] Deol AK, Fleming FM, Calvo-Urbano B, Walker M, Bucumi V, Gnandou I, et al. Schistosomiasis—Assessing progress toward the 2020 and 2025 global goals. The New England Journal of Medicine. 2019;**381**:2519-2528. DOI: 10.1056/NEJMoa1812165

[6] Salari P, Furst T, Knopp S, Utzinger J, Tediosi F. Cost of interventions to control schistosomiasis: A systematic review of the literature. PLoS Neglected Tropical Diseases. 2020;**14**:1-23. DOI: 10.1371/journal.pntd.0008098

[7] PAHA. Neglected Infectious Diseases in Amarica: Success Stories and Innovation to Reach the Neediest. Washington, DC: Pan American Health Organization (PAHA); 2016

[8] Nicolls DJ, Weld LH, Schwartz E, Reed C, von Sonnenburg F, Freedman DO, et al. Characteristics of schistosomiasis in travelers reported to the GeoSentinel surveillance network 1997-2008. The American Journal of Tropical Medicine and Hygiene. 2008;**79**:729-734

[9] https://apps.who.int/neglected_diseases/ntddata/sch/sch.html [Accessed: June 6, 2022]

[10] Christopherson JB. The curative dose of antimony tartrate in schistosomiasis (bilharzia disease). BMJ. 1923;**2**(3287):1254-1255. DOI: 10.1136/bmj.2.3287.1254

[11] WHO. Schistosomiasis: progress report 2001-2011 and strategic plan 2012-2020. Assembly WHO. Elimination of schistosomiasis. WHO

[12] Stothard JR, Campbell SJ, Osei-Atweneboana MY, Durant T, Stanton MC, Biritwum N-K, et al. Towards interruption of schistosomiasis transmission in sub-Saharan Africa: Developing an appropriate environmental surveillance framework to guide and to support 'end game' interventions. Infectious Diseases of Poverty. 2017;**6**:10. DOI: 10.1186/s40249-016-0215-9

[13] King CH, Bertsch D. Historical perspective: Snail control to prevent schistosomiasis. PLoS Neglected Tropical Diseases. 2015;**9**:e0003657. DOI: 10.1371/journal.pntd.0003657

[14] Sokolow SH, Wood CL, Jones IJ, Swartz SJ, Lopez M, Hsieh MH, et al. Global assessment of schistosomiasis control over the past century shows targeting the snail intermediate

host works best. PLoS Neglected Tropical Diseases. 2016;**10**:e0004794. DOI: 10.1371/journal.pntd.0004794

[15] Kamel B, Laidemitt MR, Lu L, Babbitt C, Weinbaum OL, Mkoji GM, et al. Detecting and identifying *Schistosoma* infections in snails andaquatic habitats: A systematic review. PLOS Neglected Tropical Diseases. 2021;**15**(3):e0009175. DOI: 10.1371/journal.pntd.0009175

[16] Carvalho OS, Jannoti-Passos LK, Caldeira RL. Importância Epidemiológica e biologia molecular aplicada ao estudo dos moluscos do gênero Biomphalaria. In: Carvalho OS, Coelho PMZ, Lenz HL, editors. Schistosoma mansoni e Esquistossomose: Uma Visão Multidiciplinar. Rio de Janeiro: Fiocruz; 2008. pp. 311-345. DOI: 10.1590/1676-0611-BN-2020-0975

[17] Palasio RGS. Estudo da variabilidade genética e morfológica de Biomphalaria tenagophila Orbigny 1835 (Gastropda, Planorbidae) procedente do Vale do Rio Ribeira do Iguape e do Litoral Norte do Estado de Sao Paulo [Projeto de Mestrado]. São Paulo: UNICAMP; 2011

[18] Tuan R, Ohlweiler FP, Palasio RGS, Zanna RD, Guimaraes MCA. Pattern of genetic divergence of mitochondrial DNA sequences in Biomphalaria tenagophila complex species based on barcode and morphological analysis. In: Rokni MB, editor. Schistosomiasis. Intech; 2012. pp. 293-309. DOI: 10.5772/25550. Available from: https://www.intechopen.com/chapters/25979

[19] Rudge JW, Carabin H, Balolong E, Tallo V Jr, Shrivastava J, Lu D, et al. Population genetics of *Schistosoma japonicum* within the Philippines suggest high levels of transmission between humans and dogs. PLoS Neglected Tropical Diseases. 2008;**2**(11):e340. DOI: 10.1371/journal.pntd.0000340

[20] Baidikul V, Upatham ES, Kruatrachue M, Viyanant V, Vichasri S, Lee P &; Chantanawat R. Study on *Schisto-soma sinensium* in Fang District, Chiangmai Province, Thailand; South East Asian Journal of Tropical Medicine and Public Health. 1984;**15**:141-147

[21] Lockyer AE, Olson PD, Ostergaard P, Rollinson D, Johnston DA, Attwood SW, et al. The phylogeny of the Schistosomatidae based on three genes with emphasis on theinterrelationships of *Schistosoma* Weinland, 1858. Parasitology. 2003;**126**:203-224

[22] Huyse T, Webster BL, Geldof S, Stothard JR, Diaw OT, Polman K, et al. Bidirectional introgressive hybridization between a cattle and human schistosome species. PLoS Pathogens. 2009;**5**(9):e1000571. DOI: 10.1371/journal.ppat.1000571

[23] Webster BL, Diaw OT, Seye MM, Webster JP, Rollinson D. Introgressive hybridization of *Schistosoma haematobium* group species in Senegal: Species barrier break down between ruminant and human schistosomes. PLoS Neglected Tropical Diseases. 2013;7:e2110. DOI: 10.1371/journal.pntd.0002110

[24] Campa P, Develoux M, Belkadi G, Magne D, Lame C, Carayon MJ, et al. Chronic Schistosoma mekongi in a traveler--a case report and review of the literature. Journal of Travel Medicine. 2014;**21**:361-363. DOI: 10.1111/jtm.12137

[25] Ross AG, Vickers D, Olds GR, Shah SM, McManus DP. Katayama syndrome. Lancet. 2007;7:218-224

[26] Tanoue M, Hirabayashi Y, Ikeuchi H. Global-scale river fiood vulnerability

in the last 50 years. Scientific Reports. 2016;**6**(36021):19. DOI: 10.1038/srep36021

[27] Rossati A. Global warming and its health impact. International Journal of Occupational and Environmental Medicine. 2017;**8**:7-20. DOI: 10.15171/ijoem.2017.963

[28] Cao C, Li S, Zhou X. Impact of schistosomiasis transmission by catastrophic flood damage and emergency response in China. Chinese Journal of Schistosomiasis Control. 2016;**28**:618-623. DOI: 10.16250/j.32.1374.2016215

[29] Yang M, Tan H, Zhou Y, Tang G, Li P, Yun C, et al. Quantitative study on human water contact during disaster year in endemic region of *schistosomiasis japonica*. Chinese Journal of Schistosomiasis Control. 2002;**14**:109-114

[30] Zhou Y, Liu Y, Wu W. Strengthen China's flood control. Nature. 2016;**536**:396. DOI: 10.1038/536396e

[31] Chen W, Yang X, Huang X, Zhang Y, Cai S, Liu J, et al. Influence of flood in 1998 on schistosomiasis epidemic. Chinese Journal of Schistosomiasis Control. 2000;**12**:202-205

[32] Diaz JH. Rodent-borne infectious disease outbreaks after flooding disasters: Epidemiology, management, and prevention. Journal of Emergency Management. 2015;**13**:459-467. DOI: 10.5055/jem.2015.0255

[33] Knight M, Wu JY, Zhou YB, Chen Y, Liang S, Li LH, et al. Three gorges dam: Impact of water level changes on the density of schistosome-transmitting snail Oncomelania hupensis in Dongting Lake area, China. PLoS Neglected Tropical Diseases. 2015;**9**:e0003882. DOI: 10.1371/journal.pntd.0003882

[34] Steinmann P, Keiser J, Bos R, Tanner M, Utzinger J. Schistosomiasis and water resources development: Systematic review, meta-analysis, and estimates of people at risk. The Lancet Infectious Diseases. 2006;**6**:411-425. DOI: 10.1016/S1473-3099(06)70521-7

[35] WHO. Tech Rep Ser. International Association For Medical Assistance To Travellers; 2002 WHO. Available from: https://www.iamat.org/ [Accessed: 2022-06-06]

[36] Crellen T, Allan F, David S, Durrant C, Huckvale T, Holroyd N, et al. Whole genome resequencing of the human parasite *Schistosoma mansoni* reveals population history and effects ofselection. Scientific Reports. 2016;**6**:20954. DOI: 10.1038/srep20954

[37] Morgan JA, DeJong RJ, Kazibwe F, Mkoji GM, Loker ES. A newly-identified lineage of Schistosoma. International Journal for Parasitology. 2003;**33**:977-985. DOI: 10.1016/s0020-7519(03)00132-2

[38] Young ND, Jex AR, Li B, Liu S, Yang L, Xiong Z, et al. Whole-genome sequence of Schistosoma haematobium. Nature Genetics. 2012;**44**(2):221-225. DOI: 10.1038/ng.1065

[39] Kane RA, Southgate VR, Rollinson D, Littlewood DT, Lockyer AE, Pagès JR. A phylogeny based on three mitochondrial genes supports the division of *Schistosoma intercalatum* into two separate species. Parasitology. 2003;**127**:131-137. DOI: 10.1017/s0031182003003421

[40] Mahmoud AAF. *Schistosomiasis*. Imperial College Press; 2001. p. 524. ISBN 978-186094-146-7 [Retrieved: 31 July 2016]

[41] Mouahid A, Théron A. Schistosoma bovis: Variability of cercarial production as related to the snail hosts: *Bulinus*

truncatus, *B. wright* and *Planorbarius metidjensis*. International Journal for Parasitology. 1987;**17**:1431-1434. DOI: 10.1016/0020-7519(87)90078-6

[42] Webster BL, Southgate VR, Littlewood DT. A revision of the interrelationships of Schistosoma including the recently described *Schistosoma guineensis*. International Journal for Parasitology. 2006;**36**:947-955. DOI: 10.1016/j.ijpara.2006.03.005

[43] Dettman CD, Higgins-Opitz SB. The infection characteristics of the antelope schistosomes, *Schistosoma margrebowiei* and *S. leiperi*, in inbred BALB/c mice and in *Mastomys coucha*. Journal of Helminthology. 1994;**1**:19-33. DOI: 10.1017/S0022149X00013420

[44] DeBont J, Vercruysse J, Sabbe F, Southgate VR, Rollinson D. Schistosoma mattheei infections in cattle: Changes associated with season and age. Veterinary Parasitology. 1995;**57**:299-307. DOI: 10.1016/0304-4017(94)00695-9

[45] Attwood SW, Fatih FA, Mondal MM, Alim MA, Fadjar S, Rajapakse RP, et al. A DNA sequence-based study of the Schistosoma indicum (Trematoda: Digenea) group: Population phylogeny, taxonomy and historical biogeography. Parasitology. 2007;**134**:14. DOI: 10.1017/S0031182007003411

[46] Agatsuma T, Iwagami M, Liu CX, Rajapakse RP, Mondal MM, Kitikoon V, et al. Affinities between Asian non-human Schistosoma species, the *S. indicum* group, and the African human schistosomes. Journal of Helminthology. 2002;**76**:7-19. DOI: 10.1079/joh200191

[47] Devkota R, Brant SV, Loker ES. A genetically distinct Schistosoma from *Radix luteola* from Nepal related to *Schistosoma turkestanicum*: A phylogenetic study of *schistosome* and snail host. Acta Tropica. 2016;**164**:45-53. DOI: 10.1016/j.actatropica.2016.08.015

[48] De Bont J, Vercruysse J, Van Aken D, Southgate VR, Rollinson D, Moncrieff C. The epidemiology of Schistosoma Spindale Montgomery, 1906 in cattle in Sri Lanka. Parasitology. 1991;**102**:237-241. DOI: 10.1017/s0031182000062545

[49] Narain K, Rajguru SK, Mahanta J. Incrimination of Schistosoma Spindale as a causative agent of farmer's dermatitis in Assam with a note on liver pathology in mice. The Journal of Communicable Diseases. 1998;**30**:1-6

[50] Attwood SW, Ibaraki M, Saitoh Y, Nihei N, Janies DA. Comparative phylogenetic studies on Schistosoma japonicum and its snail intermediate host Oncomelania hupensis: Origins, dispersal and coevolution. PLOS Neglected Tropical Diseases. 2015;**9**:e0003935. DOI: 10.1371/journal.pntd.0003935

[51] Attwood SW, Fatih FA, Upatham ES. DNA-sequence variation among Schistosoma mekongi populations and related taxa; phylogeography and the current distribution of Asian schistosomiasis. PLOS Neglected Tropical Diseases. 2008;**2**(3):e200. DOI: 10.1371/journal.pntd.0000200

[52] Attwood SW, Upatham ES, Meng XH, Qiu DC, Southgate VR. The phylogeography of Asian Schistosoma (Trematoda: Schistosomatidae). Parasitology. 2002;**125**:99-112. DOI: 10.1017/s0031182002001981

[53] Attwood SW, Brown DS, Meng XH, Southgate VR. A new species of Tricula (pomatiopsidae: Triculinae) from Sichuan province, PR China: Intermediate host of Schistosoma sinensium. Systematics and Biodiversity. 2003;**1**:109-111

[54] Kruatrachue M, Upatham ES, Sahaphong S, Tongthong T, Khunborivan V. Scanning electron microscopic study of the tegumental surface of adult Schistosoma sinensium. Southeast Asian Journal of Tropical Medicine and Public Health. 1983;**14**:427-438. DOI: 10.1017/s0031182000062545

[55] Bunnag T, Thirachandra S, Impand P, Vorasanta P, Imlarp S. Schıstosoma Incognıtum and its Zoonotıc Potentıal role In Phıtsanulok and Phıchıt Provınces, northern Thailand. Southeast Asian Journal of Tropical Medicine and Public Health. 1983;**14**:163-170

[56] Agrawal MC. *Schistosomes* and *Schistosomiasis* in South Asia. Springer; 2012. DOI: 10.1007/978-81-322-0539-5_2

[57] Tchuem Tchuenté LA, Southgate VR, Njiokou F, Njiné T, Kouemeni LE, Jourdane J. The evolution of *schistosomiasis* at Loum, Cameroon: Replacement of *Schistosoma intercalatum* by *S. haematobium* through introgressive hybridization. Transactions of the Royal Society of Tropical Medicine and Hygiene. 1997;**91**:664-665. DOI: 10.1016/s0035-9203(97)90513-7

[58] Morgan JA, DeJong RJ, Lwambo NJ, Mungai BN, Mkoji GM, Loker ES. First report of a natural hybrid between *Schistosoma mansoni* and *S. rodhaini*. The Journal of Parasitology. 2003;**89**:416-418. DOI: 10.1645/0022-3395(2003)089[0416,FROANH]2.0.CO;2

[59] Boissier J, Grech-Angelini S, Webster BL, Allienne JF, Huyse T, Mas-Coma S, et al. Outbreak of urogenital schistosomiasis in Corsica (France): An epidemiological case study. The Lancet Infectious Diseases. 2016;**16**:971-979. DOI: 10.1016/S1473-3099(16)00175-4

[60] Depaquit J, Akhoundi M, Haouchine D, Mantelet S, Izri. No limit in interspecific hybridization in *schistosomes*: Observation from a case report. Parasite. 2019;**26**:10. DOI: 10.1051/parasite/2019010

[61] World Health Organization. What Quantitative and Qualitative Methods Have Been Developed to Measure Community Empowerment at a National Level? Vol. 59. World Health Organization; 2018. Available from: https://books.google.com.tr/books?hl=tr&lr=&id=5XeyDwAAQBAJ&oi=fnd&pg=PR4&dq=Global+Health+Estimates+2016:+Deaths+by+Cause,+Age,+Sex,+by+Country+and+by+Region,+2000-2016.+Geneva,+World+Health+Organization%3B+2018.&ots=et8kJrTtpe&sig=XEzLCb_ftQDTUYO-yMB_jQb74cs&redir_esc=y#v=onepage&q&f=false [Accessed: 2022-06-06]

Chapter 6

Schistosomiasis: Discovery of New Molecules for Disease Treatment and Vaccine Development

Andressa Barban do Patrocinio

Abstract

The parasite blood flukes belonging to the genus *Schistosoma* cause schistosomiasis. Among the *Schistosoma* species that infect humans, three stand out: *Schistosoma japonicum* (*S. japonicum*), which occurs in Asia, mainly in China and the Philippines; *Schistosoma haematobium* (*S. haematobium*), which occurs in Africa; and *Schistosoma mansoni* (*S. mansoni*), which occurs in Africa and South America and the center of Venezuela (Brazil). Research has shown that these species comprise strains that are resistant to Praziquantel (PZQ), the only drug of choice to fight the disease. Moreover, patients can be reinfected even after being treated with PZQ, and this drug does not act against young forms of the parasite. Therefore, several research groups have focused their studies on new molecules for disease treatment and vaccine development. This chapter will focus on (i) parasite resistance to PZQ, (ii) molecules that are currently being developed and tested as possible drugs against schistosomiasis, and (iii) candidates for vaccine development with a primary focus on clinical trials.

Keywords: resistance of Schistosoma to PZQ, new molecules, vaccine development

1. Introduction

From the public health and socioeconomic standpoints, schistosomiasis is a parasitic disease with significant prevalence in most developing countries, and it is the second-largest neglected disease in the world [1–3]. Schistosomiasis is caused by digenean trematodes belonging to the genus *Schistosoma*. *S. mansoni*, *S. japonicum*, *S. haematobium*, *Schistosoma mekongi* (*S. mekongi*), and *Schistosoma intercalatum* (*S. intercalatum*) are the main species underlying the disease in humans. The three former species are the main causative agents of schistosomiasis [4].

The number of people living in risk areas, which cover 78 countries in tropical and subtropical regions, is greater than 700 million [5, 6]. Transmission is high or moderate in 52 of these countries (World Health Organization, 2021). More specifically, *S. mansoni* occurs in Africa and Brazil; *S. haematobium* occurs in Africa; and *S. japonicum* occurs in China, the Philippines, and some places in Indonesia. According to the WHO, there were about 10.1 million deaths due to schistosomiasis in the world in 2016 [3]. However, controlling schistosomiasis depends on the diagnosis, sanitation, and disease treatment with praziquantel (PZQ), a drug recommended by the WHO and which has been used for over 30 years [3, 7]. In 2017, 46.3% of the population was treated with PZQ; 70.8% of the treated population corresponded to school-aged children [8, 9].

S. mansoni, *S. japonicum*, and *S. haematobium* have an intricate life cycle that involves different parasite forms (miracidia, sporocysts, cercariae, schistosomula, adult worms, and eggs), in which structural and metabolic changes occur. Their life cycle requires the presence of an invertebrate host and a vertebrate host (**Figure 1**). Snails belonging to the genera *Biomphalaria*, *Bulinos*, and *Oncomelania* (intermediate hosts) release cercariae into the water, which infects the vertebrate host through the skin. In the vertebrate host, cercariae lose their tail and develop into schistosomula, which reach the pulmonary artery. In the lung, schistosomula migrate to the heart through the venous circulation. Next, schistosomula migrate to the hepatic portal system, where

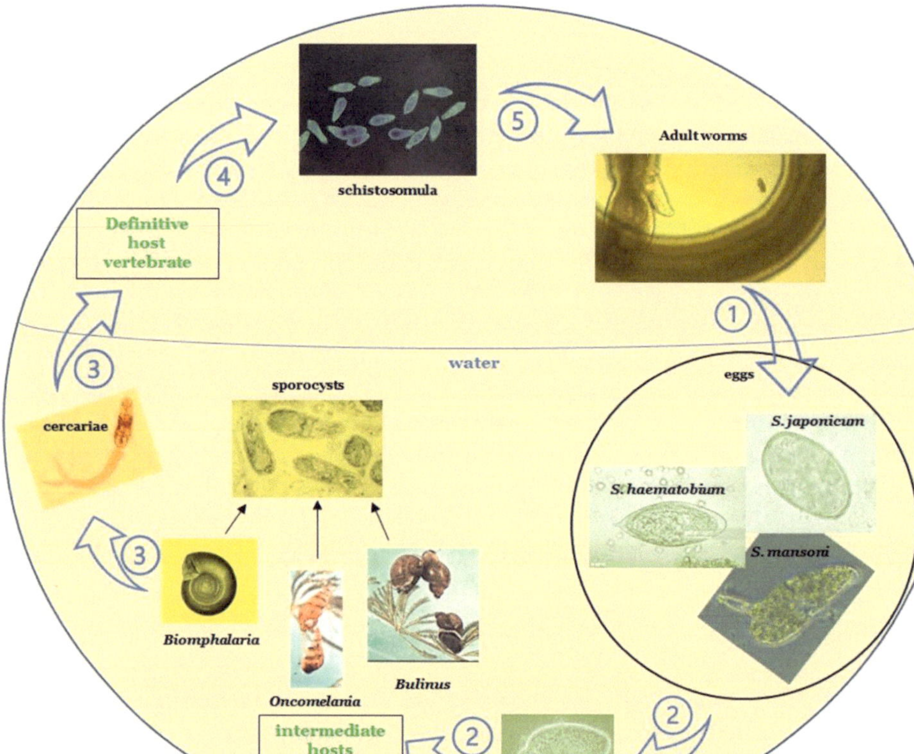

Figure 1.
S. mansoni, S. japonicum, *and* S. haematobium *life cycle—(1)* S. mansoni *and* S. japonicum *worms move to the mesenteric veins of the intestine and are lodged in different locations. Eggs are laid, and part of the eggs is released in the feces. (2) Miracidia are released from eggs into the water and infect snails (intermediate hosts). (3) Within the snail, miracidia progress through two generations of sporocysts, to become cercariae. (3) Cercariae are released from the snail and penetrate the skin of the definitive vertebrate host, releasing enzymes from glands. During penetration, cercariae lose their forked tail and become schistosomula. (4) Schistosomula migrate to the dermis veins and, upon encountering the pulmonary artery, are carried to the lungs. From the lungs, they reach the venous circulation and travel to the hepatic portal system. (5) In the hepatic portal system, schistosomula develop into adult worms, where parasite sexual maturation and pairing take place. At this time,* S. haematobium *worms are not stored in the intestine, but they inhabit the bladder pelvic venous plexus and the vesicular. Sometimes, they can be found in the rectal venules.* S. haematobium *causes urogenital schistosomiasis.*

they develop into adult worms, become sexually mature, and pair. At this time, adult *S. japonicum* and *S. mansoni* worms move to the intestine mesenteric veins and are lodged in different locations [10]—*S. japonicum* worms remain in the upper part of the vein, whereas *S. mansoni* worms remain in the lower part and close to the large intestine. Thereafter, eggs are laid, and some of them are released in the feces. In contrast, *S. haematobium* worms do not lodge in the intestine, but they inhabit the bladder pelvic venous plexus and the vesicular, where they lay eggs and cause urogenital schistosomiasis. Sometimes, *S. haematobium* worms can be found in the rectal venules. Part of the *S. haematobium* eggs is retained, whilst the other part is eliminated in the urine [11].

Schistosomiasis is characterized by two phases: acute and chronic. Symptoms of acute illness include myalgia, abdominal pain, diarrhea, fatigue, fever, and, in the case of urogenital schistosomiasis, hematuria. Diarrhea occurs in patients with a greater parasite load; abdominal pain is diffuse. In chronic intestinal schistosomiasis, symptoms are more severe. Over time, patients have diarrhea with the presence of blood in stool, anemia, and retention of eggs in the anal region, not to mention hepatosplenomegaly due to egg deposition in the liver. Hepatosplenomegaly causes granuloma (**Figure 2**) and occurs in around 10% of patients, who present periportal fibrosis with portal hypertension, ascites, and gastrointestinal varices with bleeding [12, 13]. As for urogenital schistosomiasis, it affects the urogenital system so severely that it causes fibrosis in the bladder and ureter, calcification in the urinary tract, and kidney dysfunction. The greatest concern about this urogenital disease is that it causes bladder cancer and sterility, and, in the chronic phase, patients have bladder injury [2].

The differences in schistosomiasis pathology are due to parameters such as oviposition, granuloma size, and modeling of interleukins, which depend on the parasite

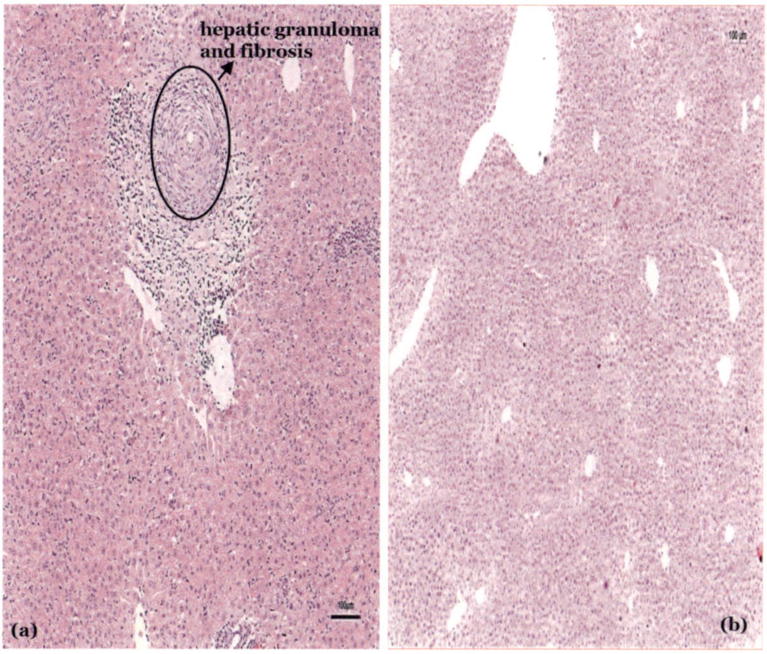

Figure 2.
Slides of (a) mouse liver infected with S. mansoni *showing hepatic granuloma and fibrosis caused by parasite eggs; purple-colored cells are eosinophils, due to inflammation in the liver (b) mouse liver not infected with* S. mansoni.

load, host's immunological profile (that is, the host's ability to respond to the parasite, whether the parasite is in the form of schistosomula, adult worms, or eggs), and parasite virulence and infectivity [14]. Therefore, the parasite and host interact in a co-evolutionary and complex way (interplay) that interferes with disease transmission potential and pathology [2].

Worm maturation requires that host-derived signals be translated, to generate adaptive and innate immune responses. Much research is still needed to unravel the interrelationship of *Schistosoma* with the immune system during worm development, maturation, pairing, and oviposition [15]. After worm couples are paired and oviposition starts, the host responds strongly to the eggs. Immediately after deposition, the eggs are surrounded by cells and proteins from the host's homeostatic system, including plasma proteins called egg-laying factors, von Willebrand factors, fibrin, and fibrinogen [15].

When it comes to schistosomiasis, egg antigens are the major problem: they are antigenic structures that secrete various toxic substances, the main one being SEA (Soluble Eggs Antigens). These toxic substances elicit the complex and multifactorial response in the mammalian host's innate immune system [15]. The acute condition of the disease is characterized by the lesion around the eggs, with the release of interferon-γ and IL-10 by macrophages and IL-12 by dendritic cells [12]. Later, another eggshell protein, ω-1, is internalized in dendritic cells, directing the Th2 response and lowering IL-12 secretion [16]. However, this does not occur in infections caused by *S. haematobium* (urogenital schistosomiasis) because the female worm does not encode this eggshell protein [2].

Thus, these parasites activate the immune system and form the highly organized granuloma that is wrapped by the Th2 immune cells, namely macrophages, eosinophils, and cells that secrete cytokines of numerous types, including IL-2, IL-4, IL-13, and IL-5, which are surrounded by stromal cells and fibroblasts. In the case of *S. haematobium*, the main interleukin is IL-5, and the fibrous granuloma has a lot of collagen and eosinophils. Urinary eosinophilia occurs because these cells release toxic substances such as eosinophilic cationic protein, neurotoxin, and granulomatous protein [2, 12].

During infection with *S. mansoni* or *S. haematobium*, IL-13 production by the vertebrate host makes it susceptible to infection—antigens released by the eggs promote a polarized Th2-type response, with fibrosis developing around the eggs due to the release of transforming growth factor (TGF)-β [17].

In the infection period, there is a balance between the Th2 and Th1 responses. The Th2 anti-inflammatory effects control the immunopathology caused by the Th1 response [18]. In *S. mansoni*-infected mice, the Th2 response is epigenetically controlled and modulates dendritic cells and macrophages, as well as Th2 cells [2]. Recently, studies have been carried out to understand the molecular relationship between parasites and hosts. Genome integrity is essential for host cells, organisms, and species survival. Hence, errors in genome checkpoints trigger cellular apoptosis to eliminate the altered cell. However, pathogens can alter these pathways by manipulating both chromatin repair and cell signaling pathways. For this to happen, pathogens produce genotoxins and oncoproteins that modify the host's epigenetic programs and influence metabolism. For this reason, they are called epigenators [19].

The Th2 response is crucial for granuloma maintenance and host survival. Proteins such as Cyclophilin A and lysophosphatidylserine (LPS), excreted from worms, can modulate the dendritic cell function, causing IL-10 to expand and activating regulatory T cells. The role of small fatty acid chains (SFACs) excreted by worms in regulating immune response is not yet known, but LPS and SCFA can modify the TLR2 signaling pathway in dendritic cells, altering maturation and regulatory T cell activation [15]. In children infected with *S. haematobium* in Uganda, regulatory B cells have been shown to induce T cells to secrete IL-10; however, in a study with Kenyan children, TNF-alpha has been correlated with inflammation and low IL-10 levels [2].

Several studies have reported that the host's immune response plays a role in PZQ effectiveness. Studies using 0-, 1-, and 3-day *S. japonicum* schistosomula have shown that the percentage of surface-exposed antigens is 86.4%, 55.2%, and 3.9%, respectively. Resistance to PZQ (PZQ-R) in these stages has been related to the antigenic composition on the tegument surface, and *in vitro* research carried out with young *S. mansoni* and *S. japonicum* larvae (3, 7 and 14 days of maturity) has demonstrated that they are resistant to PZQ [20]. Currently, PZQ is the only drug of choice against schistosomiasis. Studies have indicated that some *S. mansoni* and *S. japonicum* strains are resistant to PZQ even in the adult worm stages, as seen from the many cases of reinfected patients following multiple PZQ administrations. This situation calls for the study of new therapies, such as drugs and vaccines [21].

2. Praziquantel and schistosomiasis

The WHO has planned strategies to control schistosomiasis through PZQ administration in endemic areas where the disease is highly prevalent, mainly in Africa, in regions such as the Nile Delta, Côte d'Ivoire, Mayuge District, and Uganda. These strategies have shown that the prevalence of morbidity due to *S. mansoni* and *S. hematobium* may originate from PZQ-R and parasite-host-drug interactions, especially in areas with longer history of PZQ treatment [2, 9].

Nevertheless, the greatest PZQ-R has been detected in parasite strains maintained in the laboratory. After the passage of *S. mansoni* in seven mouse generations treated with PZQ subdoses, resistance emerged. In infections with a single *S. mansoni* sex, resistance was greater than in infections with two sexes of the parasite. This fact was later analyzed in a group of human volunteers, infected with cercariae of a single sex and treated with PZQ at the usual dose of 40 mg/kg for 12 weeks. After treatment, parasites were detected in 43% of the volunteers [9, 22]. Despite the greater PZQ-R found in the laboratory, the fact that a single drug exists for treating a certain disease must be considered seriously because variations arise from both resistant strains of disease-causing microorganisms and resistant tumorigenic cells.

PZQ has a series of pharmacological and pharmaceutical limitations that are often disregarded because the effectiveness of oral, single-dose treatment has cure rates between 50 and 90%, whether for single- or mixed-species infections [13, 23, 24]. Regarding pharmacology, PZQ exhibits suboptimal pharmacokinetics with high intra- and inter-individual variability and extensive first-pass hepatic metabolism, which results in low oral bioavailability [25]. The PZQ mechanism of action is still poorly understood, but it seems to affect Ca^{2+} absorption through calcium channel opening, which interferes with muscle contraction and leads to antigens being present in the tegument [26]. Furthermore, PZQ is only effective against adult parasites; that is, it has no antiparasitic action against schistosomula. Thus, even during treatment, immature parasites develop into mature adult worms and continue to generate morbidity in reinfected patients [27, 28]. Schistosomiasis treatment with PZQ alone increases the possibility of resistance and hence treatment failure, especially in areas where infection occurs massively [13, 29]. Academically, resistance to any drug is defined as hereditary sensitivity acquired by a living organism; that is, it is transmitted between generations [9].

One of the consequences of PZQ-R is the increasing reproduction rate of parasites that survive treatment with PZQ. One of the possible explanations for this fact is that parasites have drug-resistant alleles, which are passed from generation to generation and are related to virulence [2].

Moreover, intergeneric, interspecies, and intraspecies interactions may occur because hosts are usually infected with more than one *Schistosoma* species; for example, *S. mansoni* and *S. haematobium*. In the case of mixed infections, patient's morbidity due to hepatomegaly is lower because *S. haematobium* males recruit *S. mansoni* females from the portal vein to the vesicle plexus, where interspecies crossing takes place, with a greater number of eggs being laid in the urogenital tract [2]. Research has shown that patients infected with *S. mansoni* only have comorbidity in the bladder, which once again demonstrates an interaction between species and genetic variability and shows that the cure rate is lower in these patients than in patients infected with a single parasite species. This situation culminates in interspecies gene hybridization, with new genes being introduced. Consequently, new strains with greater transmission potential arise, making the disease difficult to control. This fact has been confirmed by genotypic analysis of *S. mansoni* schistosomula collected from patients in Senegal, who presented allelic variation at the locus L46951, where genes that transcribe mRNAs encoding proteins linked to egg production and fecundity are located. This allelic variation was increased in this lineage [2, 30].

Even the same parasite species have distinct lineages presenting greater or lesser infectivity and transmission in different endemic regions of Africa. This is due to genetic mutations caused by several factors, including environmental changes in both geographic regions and PZQ-R [30], which promote epigenetic changes in the parasite. Epigenetics is related to changes in gene expression while the DNA sequence remains unaltered. Epigenetics is one of the main regulatory systems of post-translational modifications (PTMs) in histones, which are proteins that form a unit called nucleosome [31].

In eukaryotes, chromatin is made up of genomic DNA (gDNA), RNA, and proteins. The main proteins are called histones, which are divided into isoforms. The main isoforms are H2A, H2B, H3, and H4, which form octamers around gDNA, consisting of two dimers, H3-H4 and H2A-H2B. At physiological pH, histones bear a positive charge and interact with the negative charge on gDNA, thereby constituting the basic unit called nucleosome, which closes the DNA structure. The nucleosome structure allows the terminal carbon and nitrogen tails (C-t and N-t, respectively) of these proteins to undergo PTMs [31]. The PTMs of these proteins include lysine acetylation and methylation (K), serine/threonine phosphorylation (Ser/Thr), and ubiquitination, among others. These PTMs are covalent modifications, and their set is called the "histone code" [32], with more than one PTM occurring in a histone molecule.

3. Parasite epigenetics interferes with the host's immune response

Metabolic alterations and environmental changes (nutritional deprivation, temperature, and chemical agents) generate a stressful environment for living organisms. The stress mechanism is activated and causes activation of other regulatory mechanisms, including gene transcription, which generates an "epigenetic memory" in response to stress. This mechanism has been detected in *S. cerevisiae* and *C. elegans* [31–34].

Studies have been carried out to understand how the molecular relationship between parasites and hosts works. Genome integrity is essential for host cells, organisms, and species survival. Thus, errors in genome checkpoints trigger cellular apoptosis, to eliminate the altered cell. However, pathogens can alter these pathways by manipulating both chromatin repair and cell signaling pathways. For this to happen, pathogens produce genotoxins and oncoproteins that modify the host's epigenetic programs; that is, DNA expression, which consequently influences metabolism by altering the proteins that will be expressed. For this reason, pathogens are called epigenators. Some intracellular parasites such as *Theileria parva* and *Theileria annulata* encode proteins that manipulate the host's intracellular pathways. For example, toxoplasma secretes the GRA16 protein, which is exported to the nucleus and interferes with the p53 protein pathway "checkpoint." Studies have reported that *Leishmania* prevents or modulates the host's immune response because it can methylate the macrophage DNA cytosine residue and silence immune response genes like calcium, JAK/STAT, MAPK, mTOR, and Notch [19, 35].

Some studies are being carried out on *S. mansoni*. As this parasite changes stages, metabolic and molecular alterations occur, naturally generating stress. In addition to environmental changes, there are nutritional differences between one environment and the other because the different *S. mansoni* forms pass through two hosts, a mammal and a snail of the genus *Biomphalaria,* not to mention water as an infection route. The parasite is suitable for diverse environments due to its hereditary phenotypic capacity [36]. Epigenetic regulation, which is linked to hereditary phenotypic capacity, occurs through "readers," "erasers," and "writers," which respectively correspond to proteins with certain domains that recognize histone tagging; enzymes that remove histone labeling, such as histone deacetylases (HDACs); and histone demethylases, which promote both histone and gDNA labeling [37].

The *S. mansoni* genome comprises 363 megabases; 11,000 genes of these megabases encode proteins. Analysis of the parasite genome predicts methylation of 25 "readers," 13 "erasers," and 26 "writers." All this machinery is regulated during parasite development, which makes it a target for the discovery of new drugs [36]. When the parasite changes stages, there are molecular changes and alterations in the signaling pathways, which are accompanied by "histone code" remodeling. A study using chromatin immunoprecipitation/sequencing (CHIP-Seq) and RNAseq from the cercaria to the adult worm stages has shown changes in H3K4 and H3K27 methylation. Besides that, when cercariae change to schistosomula, H3K27me3/H3K9me3 is demethylated, consequently activating gene replication and increasing H3K9 methylation and acetylation above and below the transcription site. H3K4me3 is a constant mark during the parasite life cycle; i.e., it does not vary. Bivalent H3K4 and H3K27 trimethylation at transcription initiation sites is a hallmark of cercariae, where these sites exist at a higher level. However, this feature is also present in primary sporocysts and adult worms and increases from miracidium to primary sporocysts, with H3K27 being a necessary hallmark in life cycle progression. H4K20me1 is also a strong marker in cercariae [38, 39].

Given that the parasite can act as an epigenator, to modify the host's immune response to the disease, it is extremely important to know how chromatin epigenetic regulation occurs upon changes in temperature, pH, osmolarity, and physical and biochemical signals in *Schistosoma* species and upon alterations in the parasite/host relationship. The first question is about how the parasite manages to survive an average of 5 years in its definitive host; there are cases in which it can interact for up to 10 years [13]. The main barrier to parasite action is the host's immune response to schistosomula, eggs, and adult worms.

With respect to *S. mansoni* schistosomula and adult worms, the parasite-host interface is still poorly studied. A large immunological barrier is known to exist when schistosomula infect the mammalian host, as previously mentioned. From the moment schistosomula leave the skin until they reach the host's venous system and migrate to the lung, 3 days elapse. Eight days after infection, schistosomula reach the portal vein system, with few morphological changes. In this life cycle stage, the parasite tegument surface is modified through acquisition of molecules from the host. This stimulates receptors on inner membranes, aiding parasite development and escape from the host's immune response. Upon reaching the portal system, parasite cell proliferation and cell biomass increase significantly, promoting morphological alterations [40].

New drugs or vaccines against schistosomiasis must be discovered—*Schistosoma* is a complex organism, which makes the discovery of new substances that can halt these parasites difficult. This is one of the reasons why PZQ has been used to treat schistosomiasis for 40 years. To overcome this issue, several investigations have been carried out to study PZQ-resistant *Schistosoma* species strains [9, 26, 41].

4. Developing vaccines and new drugs to treat schistosomiasis

Research aimed at discovering a vaccine against schistosomiasis involves selecting possible parasite antigens that are expressed in the intra-mammalian stages. These antigens activate the host's immune system, forming memory cells. Reaction of immunoglobulins IgA, IgG, and IgM excreted by immune system cells is analyzed by the Enzyme-linked Immunosorbent Assay (ELISA) reaction with antigens from *Schistosoma* species adult worms, schistosomula, and eggs [42]. In immunology, ELISA is widely used for quantifying and detecting antigens and antibodies. The assay is performed in a high adhesion 96-well plate, and the antibody that binds to a specific antigen is added to the plate. Then, a chemiluminescent substrate is added, and the amount of antibody produced as a response to the studied antigen is detected through the color intensity of the sample in relation to a standard curve (Alice V. Lin).

As for the discovery of new drugs, it involves substances that act against tegumentary proteins or proteins that are linked to parasite metabolism. The initial tests on the investigated substances are called *in vitro* tests: these tests are carried out on parasites in culture medium containing the evaluated substance. Biochemical tests (**Figure 3**) are conducted to investigate the possible mechanism of action of the evaluated substance. Examples of such tests include proteins involved in autophagy and apoptosis as well as scanning and transmission electron microscopy for analysis of cellular structures and tegumentary injury and verification of changes in parasite biology that lead to parasite death [43–51].

After the first *in vitro* phase for investigation of target proteins in the parasite (for vaccine development) or new molecules (for drug development) is performed, preclinical tests are accomplished in animals (mice, rabbits, or baboons). Later, clinical trials (divided into phases I, II, III, and IV) in humans are carried out. Phase I aims to generate safety and efficacy data for both vaccines and new drugs; phase II aims to establish vaccine immunogenicity; phase III demonstrates the effectiveness of the vaccine or drug and promotes their approval by regulatory bodies, such as the FDA; and phase IV is when the vaccine is made available to the population.

"In 2016, Science ranked the schistosomiasis vaccine as one of the 10 vaccines that urgently need to be developed to make a significant impact on reducing the global

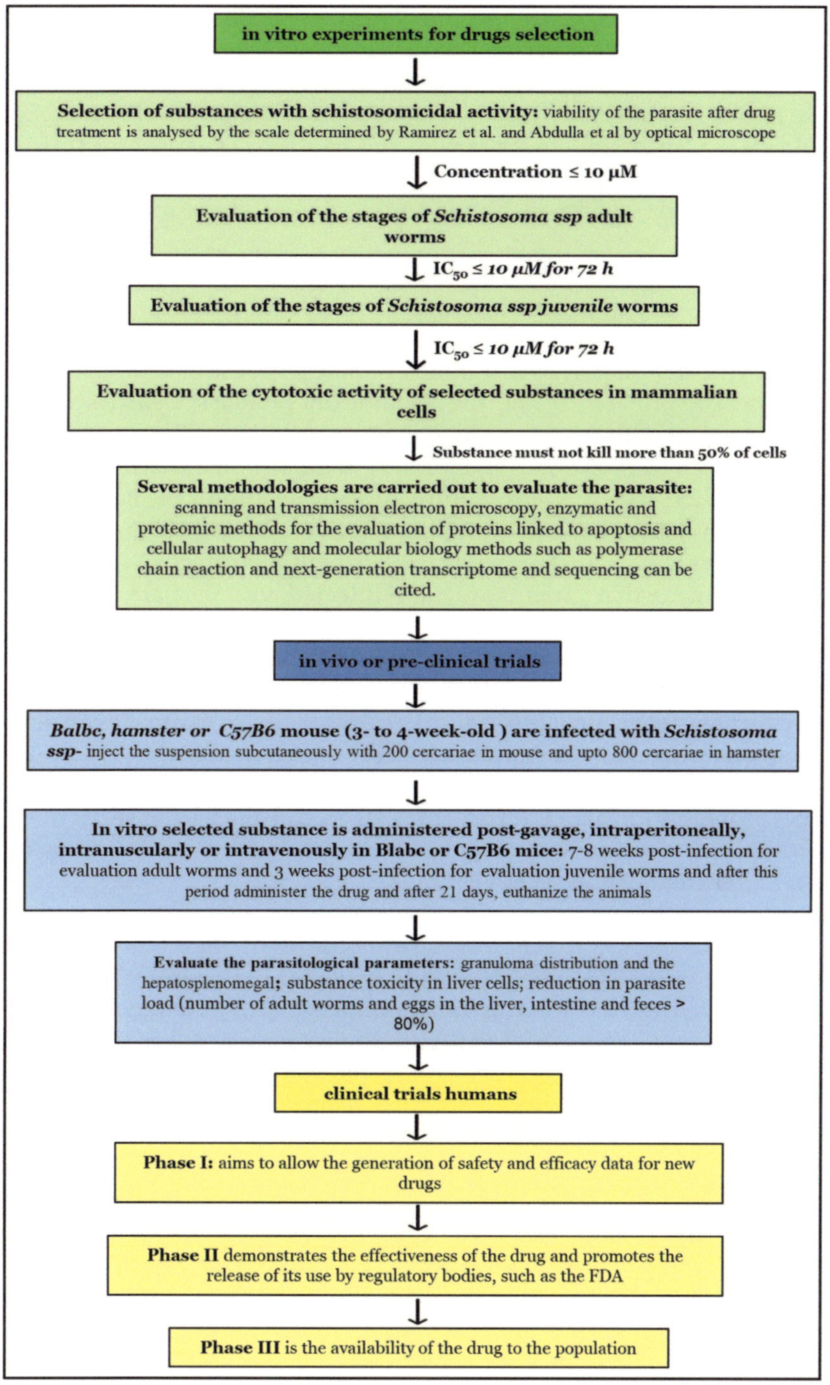

Figure 3.
Scheme for discovering new drugs to treat schistosomiasis. The discovery of a new medication for schistosomiasis takes a long time, 10 years or more. The steps involve in vitro *research when cultures of the parasites are treated with the study drug. If the parasite dies or if changes in the tegument and internal structures of the parasite occur, as detected by the methodologies mentioned in the diagram, tests on mammalian cells are performed to evaluate the toxicity of the substance. After this evaluation,* in vivo *tests are carried out. When the parasite load decreases by more than 80% and toxicity to liver cells is low, the substance is directed to clinical trials to determine whether there is a schistosomicidal effect, and if there are side effects in humans (Flavio C. Lombardo).*

burden of diseases." In 2013, a meeting with 70 experts from the Bill and Melinda Gates Foundation considered that an effective vaccine against schistosomiasis should reduce the parasite load and pathology caused by eggs by 75%; in other words, granulomas in the liver and urogenital tract should be reduced. In addition, an effective vaccine should elicit adaptive immune response and be effective against the three main *Schistosoma* species (*S. mansoni*, *S.* haematobium, and *S. japonicum*) or at least against the two former species, which cohabit the same regions of disease infestation [52].

4.1 Vaccines

New vaccines are developed by using recombinant proteins, and their effectiveness is tested by verifying whether they generate an immune response when applied to mammals. For the schistosomiasis vaccine, the recombinant protein system has proteins that are part of the surface of the parasite and that are secreted by it. These proteins have previously been selected by proteomics and transcriptome and analyzed *in vitro*. They are expressed in HEK-293 cells in *in vitro* culture. After evaluation of the humoral immune response by ELISA, preclinical and clinical assays are performed (**Figure 4**).

Developing a vaccine, which does not need to be 100% effective against schistosomiasis, will ensure that patients are not reinfected with the parasite, especially in endemic areas where morbidity is high. If this goal is reached, disease control is achieved [11]. However, discovering a vaccine is difficult because the parasite can escape the host's immune system [53]. This escape can occur through epigenetic changes in the parasite genome [40, 54, 55]. Additionally, the parasite can act as an epigenitor, interfering with the expression of proteins linked to the vertebrate host's immune system through genotoxins, also called bioactive molecules. Genotoxins can be enzymes or inhibitors that modify histone PTM, causing a balance between resisting reinfection and controlling the immune response (e.g., in relation to eggs retained in the liver) after treatment with PZQ [13].

The possibility that *Schistosoma ssp* act as an epigenitor comes from research showing that *Schistosoma*-specific proteins play an essential role in their hosts' biological processes. In this context, 100 biomolecules of great importance for helminth survival have been researched and identified as vaccine targets [56, 57]. No vaccine against schistosomiasis has been approved, but these bioactive molecules have been identified by new techniques, including genomics, transcriptomics, microarrays, proteomics, and immunological profiling [57]. Immune response against *Schistosoma* species is multifactorial and complicated because it involves IgE and several cytokines of the immune system [13].

Vaccines that are being tested in humans include Sh28GST (Bilvax-Phase III), which offers 30–60% protection; Smp80 (phase I), which offers 30–70% protection; Smp14 (phase I), which offers 50–68% protection; and SmTPS1 and Sm-TSP-2 (phase I), which offer 65–69% protection [56, 57].

Techniques for producing vaccines with recombinant proteins are described below for further understanding of their tests. As an example, we will mention a vaccine that is in the test phase and which is based on the parasite protein p80, called calpain. The parasite protein p80 is present in the inner membrane of the tegument of adult worms and other *S. mansoni*, *S. hamatobium*, and *S. japonicum* stages. This protein accelerates the synthesis of proteins of signaling pathways, which in turn accelerates tegumentar membrane surface renewal and evasion of the host's immune response [57].

Preclinical trials with many types of the Sm-p80-based vaccine, tested in mice infected with *S. mansoni*, have shown protection and reduced parasite load.

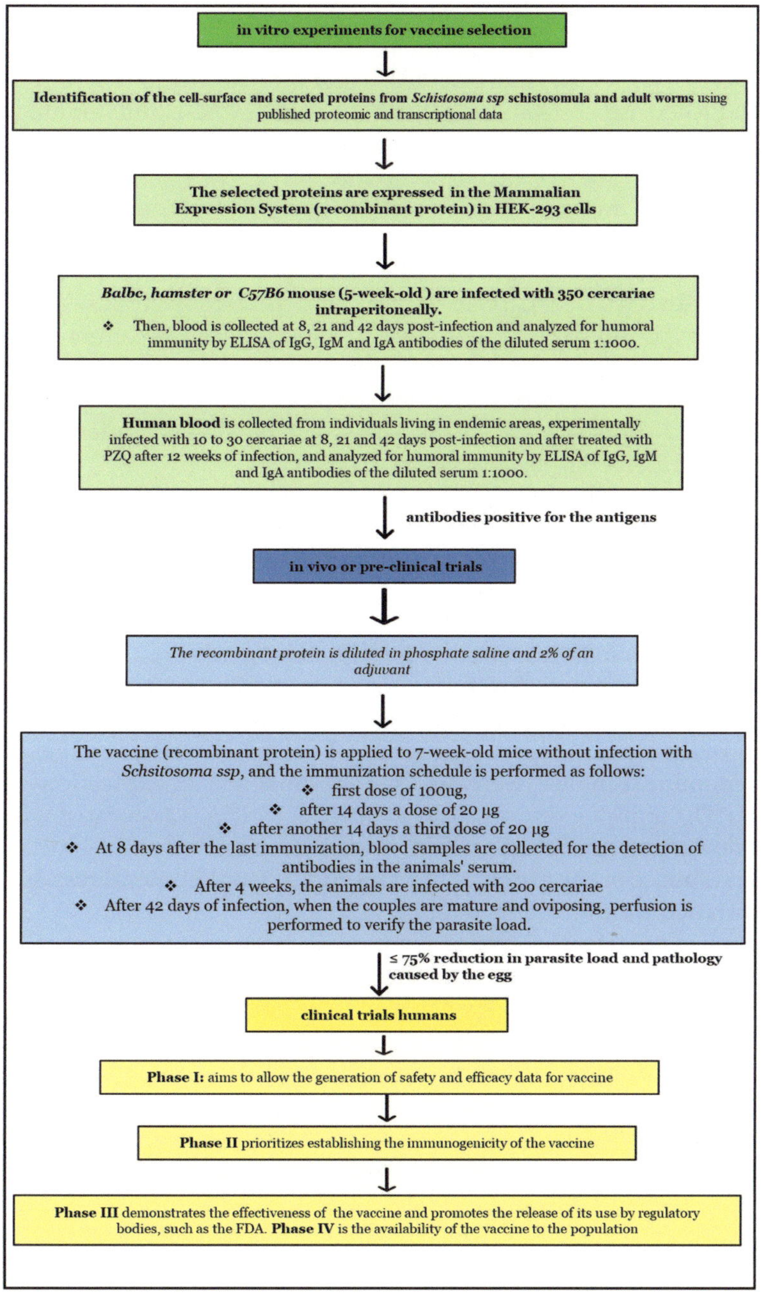

Figure 4.
Scheme for discovering schistosomiasis vaccine. Vaccine development involves several steps including in vitro, *and clinical screening. The flowchart of how this process is carried out is outlined in the figure.*

The Deoxyribonucleic Acid-based vaccine (p80-pcDNA3 DNA) reduced oviposition by 84% and promoted humoral immune response (IgG2a and IgG2b Ab) in animals and mice vaccinated with either purified Sm-p80 or p80-pcDNA3 DNA; mononuclear macrophages secreted high IFN-γ and IL-2 levels (Th1 response). Then, the Sm-p80 DNA-based vaccine was tested in baboons, which had parasite-specific IgG activation.

Protection was detected between 5 and 8 years after vaccination [42, 57, 58]. For this trial, recombinant Sm-p80 (*S. mansoni*) (Sm-p80 + GLA-SE) was encoded from the complete Sm-p80 sequence in pCold II vector for transformation into *E. coli BL21* (DE3). Protein expression was confirmed by SDS-PAGE and immunoblotting. Initially, three different adjuvants were tested for vaccine formulation; the best adjuvant was the stable oil-in-water emulsion (GLA-SE), a TLR4 glucopyranosyl lipid A agonist. To verify the immunization strategy, 30 baboons were used: 15 controls were intramuscularly injected with 5 µg of GLA-SE, while 15 baboons were intramuscularly immunized with 25 µg of rSm-p80 in 5 µg of GLA-SE. After vaccination, the baboons were infected with cercariae. Baboons were used in this study because their immune system resembles the human immune system. The baboons were immunized with a higher dose of vaccine (250 µg), in a total of three doses (0, 4, and 8 weeks) from primary vaccination to the third boost, and they had their parasitological parameters monitored to verify disease progression. Then, each baboon was infected with 1000 *S. mansoni* cercariae 12 weeks post-vaccination [59].

After vaccination and infection with cercariae, the livers of the mice and baboons were removed, and transcriptome was performed by using RNAseq. This technique is used for sequencing and expression analysis of the mRNA set. In the case described here, this technique was used to analyze which host genes linked to the immune system would be active during the development of protection due to vaccination. RNAseq analysis of mouse liver showed high expression of genes linked to coding of innate immune response proteins; inflammatory cytokines such as IL-1, IL-15, IL-18, and the TNF superfamily; interferon; and complement factors. In addition, high IL-27 levels, related to IL-12 involved in CD4+ T cell proliferation and genes related to adaptive immune response, were detected. In baboon liver, expression of mRNA related to the Th1 immune response was identified. This was associated with differentiation and development of T cells, which are memory cells of paramount importance for immune response in the presence of parasite. CD8 and humoral responses with B cell differentiation were also detected [59].

When applied to mice, the vaccine mentioned above provided promising results with high IgM, IgA, and IgG levels and protection for up to 60 weeks after it was administered. At the end of the experiments, the recombinant vaccine showed between 30% and 70% protection. The next test, carried out on baboons, provided around 50% protection and 100% reduction in eggs in the liver and intestine, which should prevent disease transmission [56, 59]. The same vaccine was also administered to hamsters and baboons infected with *S. haematobium*, resulting in lower oviposition by female parasites and, consequently, reduced number of eggs in the tissues and a balance between the Th1 and Th2 responses [57].

For *S. haematobium*, a recombinant vaccine has been monovalently produced from the enzyme glutathione (S)-transferase (Sh28GST). The protein 28GST has been identified in the three main *Schistosoma* species, in the tegument, parenchyma, and genital organs of adult parasites and in schistosomula. As a vaccine, Sm28GST was also expressed as a recombinant protein in *E. coli* and purified (rSm28GST/BCG). In pre-clinical studies carried out in mice, the immunological response elicited by the vaccine encompassed the immunoglobulins IgG1/IgG2a and IgG2b. Sh28GS (*S. haematobium*) promoted cross-protection not only against *S. haematobium* but also against other *Schistosoma* species. Immunizations with rSh28GST in adult males (phase Ia) showed that the vaccine had no systemic toxicity or cross-reaction with human GST. The volunteers showed high levels of specific neutralizing antibodies against the parasite, especially after the third dose. In the screening phase Ib, performed with children, satisfactory results were obtained: IgG1, IgG2, IgG3, and Th2 cytokines (IL-5, IL-10, and IL-13) were produced [56].

Tetrapanin proteins (TSP) are transmembrane proteins of the tegument detected at all stages of the parasite life cycle. TSP is exposed to the host's immune system. The main TSP is Sm-TSP-2, which has been used for testing vaccine development. In animal models, the recombinant Sm-TSP-2 vaccine protected the animals and decreased the parasite load and eggs in the liver. The neutralization response of the animals to the vaccine involved IgG1, IgG2 Abs., and IgG3. Later, a study was carried out with the recombinant vaccine, Recombinant Sm-TSP-2 vaccine formulated on aluminum hydroxide adjuvant (Sm-TSP-2/Al), in infected volunteers from non-endemic areas. The volunteers responded with increased IgG production. Projects encouraged by the Sabin Institute and in support of schistosomiasis vaccines have been launched, and a new recombinant vaccine, called Sm-TSP-2/Alhydrogel, is in phase 2 clinical trials in Brazil and the USA [57].

Another vaccine, still in pre-clinical testing for *S. mansoni* and *S. japonicum*, is based on a protein called Paramyosin (Pmy, 97 kDa). Pmy, which is present in the tegument and muscle of adult worms, tegument of schistosomula, and glands of cercariae, promotes the release of enzymes that help to penetrate the vertebrate host's skin. Pmy is important for immune response evasion by the parasites given that it inhibits proteins C1 and C9 and binds to polymeric collagen and IgG, thereby inhibiting innate and acquired immune response activation through microorganism opsonization. Therefore, Pmy is linked to inhibition of host's infection and reinfection. To test the vaccine based on Pmy, Swiss mice were immunized with three doses of purified Sm97. After immunization, the sera of these animals showed high levels of humoral immune response, linked to specific anti-Sm97 IgG1 and IgG2. Moreover, the parasite load, the number of eggs in the liver, and intestine of the animals decreased. However, this vaccine did not inhibit cercaria penetration in mice infected with *S. mansoni*, but it inhibited *S. japonicum* cercaria penetration through the host's skin by 62–86%. These data led the vaccine to clinical screening phase I, carried out in 616 participants, to verify protection against *S. japonicum* reinfection. The participants' protection profiles involved IgA, IgE, and IgG activation. Studies in the clinical phase are currently underway [57, 60].

The 14-kDa protein FABP is located in the basal part of the tegument and intestinal epithelium of all the stages of the parasite life cycle, including eggs. Because *Schistosoma* species do not have the machinery to produce fatty acids, FABP is responsible for the uptake, compartmentalization, and transport of fatty acids from the vertebrate host through the tegument of the parasite to its interior. The vaccine based on this protein has been produced by using the recombinant protein (rSml4/GLA-SE). When this vaccine was applied in rabbits and mice, it reduced the *S. mansoni* load by 89% and 67%, respectively. The clinical trial phase 1, which involved 20 male volunteers from endemic areas in Brazil, showed that the vaccine, applied in three doses, was highly immunogenic and safe. The humoral immune response increased, with high levels of specific total IgG1 and IgG2, IgG3, and IgG4, and low levels of IgE, IgA, and IgM being produced. An immune response dependent on IFNγ and TNFα took place. The next step will be phase II trials in endemic areas of Brazil and Africa [56, 61].

4.2 New drugs

Molecules that alter the parasite tegument structure must be considered as possible new drugs because the tegument is essential for parasite survival in mammalian hosts: indeed, the tegument plays an important role in evading immune response and acquiring nutrients from the host [53].

To date, no new molecule has reached the clinical screening phase, but several studies are in the preclinical and *in vitro* phases. Analyses of the transcriptome; that is, the *Schistosoma* mRNA set, have led to promising new targets against the parasite [13].

Some drugs are administered to treat schistosomiasis. One example is metrifonate, which has been used to treat urogenital schistosomiasis. Nevertheless, this drug requires that several doses be administered, and it has several side effects. Another drug is Oltipraz, which acts against *S. mansoni* and *S. haematobium*. However, 2 months are necessary for the patient to be cured, so patients usually give up the treatment. This drug reduces the levels of the parasite enzyme glutathione synthase, which facilitates worm elimination by the immune system. As for niridazole, it reduces the parasite glycogen levels and degenerates the female reproductive system. It is effective *against S. haematobium*, but protection against *S. japonicum* lies between 30% and 70%. However, today patients are no longer given the drug due to side effects on both the central nervous system and heart. Another problem is that this drug is no longer effective against *S. japonicum* males. The drug oxamniquine acts on *S. mansoni* by affecting the synthesis of nucleic acids, consequently impacting DNA, RNA, and protein translation. However, oxamniquine has been used for 20 years, so *S. mansoni* has become resistant to it [26].

The association of anthelmintic drugs with antimalarials is advantageous for research aimed at discovering combinations that eliminate not only the adult stage of the parasite but also schistosomula. Drug combinations are an alternative to treatment with PZQ monotherapy [62].

Concomitant administration of OXA and PZQ to treat *S. mansoni*-infected mice has been more successful than administration of individual drugs. OXA combined with PZQ has been orally administered in children aged between 8 and 20 years infected with *S. mansoni* or *S. haematobium*, and clinical screening has been carried out. Oral administration of 15–20 mg/kg PZQ associated with OXA (7.5–10 mg/kg) reduced egg shedding by between 93% and 99% in children infected with *S. mansoni*. In children infected with *S. haematobium*, this combination did not succeed in treating urogenital schistosomiasis [62].

Drugs used for malaria treatment have been tested in association with PZQ in preclinical trials. The combination that reduced the parasite load and the number of eggs went on to the clinical phase in endemic regions of Africa and Asia, where transmission and reinfection rates are high. Various combinations have been administered to patients infected with *S. mansoni*, *S. japonicum*, or *S. haematobium*. Among these combinations, Artesunate (AS) + PZQ and Sulfamethoxypyrazine/Pyrimethamine + AS can be mentioned, none of which has provided better results than monotherapy with PZQ [62].

Mefloquine (MFQ), an antimalarial drug, has been considered the best *in vitro* tests performed against *Schistosoma*. MFQ damaged the parasite tegument, muscles, and reproductive and digestive systems. Therefore, MFQ was tested in combination with PZQ and Artemisin, to see whether these combinations would be more effective than PZQ monotherapy. Clinical trials performed on children infected with *S. mansoni* and/or *S. haematobium* showed that the combinations did not outperform PZQ monotherapy even though association with antimalarial drugs was expected to increase the action of PZQ against schistosomula.

Despite the importance of PZQ monotherapy, this drug does not treat granulomas caused by eggs in the liver. Therefore, in addition to PZQ-resistant parasite strains, changes in liver histopathology are a problem in patients with chronic disease, especially in areas where reinfection occurs [62].

Recently, researchers have studied extracts of substances of plant origin, but most studies are in the *in vitro* phase. Among the studied extracts, we can mention (−)-6,6-dinitrohinokinin (DNK), which alters the tegument of *S. mansoni* couples, separating them and reducing the number of eggs and the rate of egg development. The *in vivo* test in mice infected with *S. mansoni* and treated with DNK revealed a smaller number of eggs per gram of tissue, which consequently reduced the size of the spleen and liver; the parasite load also decreased [63]. Cramoll-1,4-lectine, isolated from *Cratylia mollis,* has been shown to have antiparasitic activity in mice infected with *S. mansoni* and treated with 7 mg/kg for 7 days. Egg excretion, worm recovery, and granulomas decreased by 80%, 20%, and 73% in these animals [64].

Among medicinal plants with high schistosomicidal activity, *Zingiber officinale* can be cited. *Zingiber* has antifungal, antibacterial, and antioxidant effects. Moreover, it acts as anthelmintic, improving granulomatous inflammation. Due to their cost-effectiveness, nanoparticles (NPs) have been used against infectious agents. NPs can enter small capillaries, which allows better absorption, entry into target tissues, and lower toxicity. *Zingiber* extract is made up of nanoparticles (GNPs) that are easy to purify, which facilitates its use. In pre-clinical trials, GNPs (5 mg/kg or 2.5 mg/kg) were orally administered 3 days/week for 5 weeks. This treatment was started 4 weeks after mice were infected with *S. mansoni*. The number of eggs in the liver was evaluated: the egg load reduced by 65%, as verified by histopathology. Furthermore, worm recovery from infected mice decreased by 60%. Scanning electron microscopy images showed changes in tegument integrity, which occurred 10 weeks post-infection and was due to the antioxidant effect, as evaluated by enzymes linked to oxidative stress. Together, these results indicated that GNPs have hepatoprotective, schistosomicidal, and antioxidant functions [65].

Due to their anti- and pro-fibrotic function, small molecules, called microRNAs (miRNAs), have been researched for schistosomiasis treatment. miRNAs are small RNAs that are not translated into proteins. They contain around 70 nucleotides and are important for cellular homeostasis: they are involved in the post-transcriptional regulation of one-third of the protein-coding genes and hence participate in the activation or inhibition of cellular processes. miRNAs have been the target of research into the therapy of diseases such as cancer, diabetes, viral diseases, and other metabolic diseases. Through molecular biology techniques, they can be detected in tissues, plasma, serum, and biological fluids. These techniques include Polymerase Chain Reaction, Microarrays, and RNA Sequencing, which together amplify nucleotides and sequence them in order to discover their sequences [66]. Therefore, several miRNAs are being studied for the therapy of diseases such as solid tumors and hematopoietic diseases. Examples of such miRNAs include MiR-34 and MRX34 (the liposomal miR-34a mimic), which are in the phase I preclinical trials [67].

Along with the genotoxins produced by the parasites, which alter the host's immune response [35], vertebrate host miRNAs play a role in the parasite-host relationship, so they have been studied as biomarkers for schistosomiasis detection and hepatic fibrosis gene therapy. Such studies are in the preclinical trial phase. Initial research has shown that miR-21 and miR-96 are involved in regulating the immune response and hence hepatic granuloma by regulation of the TGF β/SMAD pathway, linked to collagen formation. Therefore, they have a pro-fibrotic function, in contrast to miR-203-3p, which is anti-fibrotic. In the case of schistosomiasis, there are miRNAs that characterize liver changes and hepatosplenomegaly progression. Among these miRNAs, we can mention MiR-223: the serum of mice infected with *S. japonicum* showed high levels of this miRNA, which returned to normal levels after treatment with PZQ. Other miRNAs, such as miR-2c-3p, are related to fibrosis progression in mice infected with *S. japonicum*. Therapy through miRNA silencing, whose function is to decrease gene transcription of pro-fibrotic genes, is being tested in infected mice by using viral vectors such as lentiviruses and adenoviruses. The genome of these vectors has antisense sequences that can inhibit host profibrotic miRNAs. In independent experiments, the viral vectors lenti-let-7b and adeno-associated virus serotype 8 (rAAV8)-mediate (which inhibits miR-21 and miR-96) were injected into mice infected with *S. japonicum*, to slow down the collagen production activation pathway and to reduce hepatic granuloma. However, these studies are initial and further research is needed [68].

In view of what has been explained, the development of new vaccines for schistosomiasis is more advanced than the development of new drugs against this disease. As judged from the time that PZQ, the only drug of choice, has been used, developing new substances that are active against the parasite is difficult. When it comes to evading the host's immune response, *Schistosoma* species have put together a strategy to follow their cycle from schistosomula to adult worm, so that they reach oviposition while balancing the host's TH1 and Th2 immune responses. This strategy allows the parasite to survive for up to 10 years in the host. Therefore, the biological complexity of *Schistosoma* species prevents reinfections with these species from being avoided and causes the parasite to become resistant to PZQ. In conclusion, several biological molecules of the parasite (genotoxins and miRNAs, not mentioned in this chapter) interfere in the parasite-host relationship, not to mention the vertebrate host's microRNAs that alter this relationship, generating a network of molecules that interacts with each other. Furthermore, the biological complexity of the parasite involves a cycle consisting of different phases (cercariae, miracidia, eggs, adult worms, schistosomula, and daughter sporocysts) during which the parasite structure and metabolism change according to the environment in which it is inserted (that is, whether the parasite is in the intermediate or definitive host or in water).

Author details

Andressa Barban do Patrocinio
Department of Biochemistry and Immunology, Fiocruz-Bi-Institutional Translational Medicine Project, Ribeirao Preto Medical School, Ribeirao Preto, SP, Brazil

*Address all correspondence to: abarbandopatrocinio@gmail.com

References

[1] Kalantari P, Bunnell SC, Stadecker MJ. The C-type lectin receptor-driven, Th17 cell-mediated severe pathology in Schistosomiasis: Not all immune responses to helminth parasites are Th2 dominated. Frontiers in Immunology. 2019;**10**(Jan):1-7. DOI: 10.3389/fimmu.2019.00026

[2] Mawa PA, Kincaid-Smith J, Tukahebwa EM, Webster JP, Wilson S. Schistosomiasis morbidity hotspots: Roles of the human host, the parasite and their interface in the development of severe morbidity. Frontiers in Immunology. 2021;**12**(March):1-21. DOI: 10.3389/fimmu.2021.635869

[3] Silva-Moraes V, Shollenberger LM, Siqueira LMV, Castro-Borges W, Harn DA, Grenfell RFQE, et al. Diagnosis of *Schistosoma mansoni* infections: What are the choices in Brazilian low-endemic areas? Memorias Do Instituto Oswaldo Cruz. Mar 28 2019;**114**:e180478. DOI: 10.1590/0074-02760180478. PMID: 30942278, PMCID: PMC6440364

[4] Pinto-Almeida A, Mendes T, de Oliveira RN, de Andrade Penteado Corrêa S, Allegretti SM, Belo S, et al. Morphological characteristics of *Schistosoma mansoni* PZQ-resistant and -susceptible strains are different in presence of praziquantel. Frontiers in Microbiology. 2016;**7**(Apr):1-11. DOI: 10.3389/fmicb.2016.00594

[5] PAHOA. 2022. Available from: https://www3.paho.org/hq/index.php?option=com_content&view=article&id=13650:schistosomiasis-factsheet-health-workers&Itemid=40721&lang=en [Accessed: April 23, 2022]

[6] WHO. 2022. Available from: https://www.who.int/health-topics/schistosomiasis#tab=tab_1 [Accessed: April 23, 2022]

[7] Caffrey CR. Schistosomiasis and its treatment. Future Medicinal Chemistry. 2015;**9**:675-676

[8] Lima MG, Montresor LC, Pontes J, Augusto R d C, da Silva JP, Thiengo SC. Compatibility polymorphism based on long-term host-parasite relationships: Cross talking between Biomphalaria Glabrata and the trematode *Schistosoma mansoni* from endemic areas in Brazil. Frontiers in Immunology. 2019;**10**(April):328. DOI: 10.3389/fimmu.2019.00328

[9] Yu QF, Zhang JY, Sun MT, Man Man G, Zou HY, Webster JP, et al. In vivo praziquantel efficacy of *Schistosoma japonicum* over time: A systematic review and meta-analysis. Acta Tropica. 2021;**222**(March):106048. DOI: 10.1016/j.actatropica.2021.106048

[10] Kunz W. Schistosome male-female interaction: Induction of germ-cell differentiation. Trends in Parasitology. 2001;**17**(5):227-231. DOI: 10.1016/S1471-4922(01)01893-1

[11] Mcmanus DP. Schistosomiasis—From immunopathology to vaccines. Seminars in Immunopathology. 2020;**42**(3):355-371

[12] Giorgio S, Gallo-Francisco PH, Roque GAS, e Silva MF. Granulomas in parasitic diseases: The good and the bad. Parasitology Research. 2020;**119**(10):3165-3180. DOI: 10.1007/s00436-020-06841-x

[13] McManus DP, Dunne DW, Sacko M, Utzinger J, Vennervald BJ, Zhou XN. Schistosomiasis. Nature Reviews Disease Primers. 2018;**4**(1):1-19. DOI: 10.1038/s41572-018-0013-8

[14] Mota EA, Do Patrocínioid AB, Rodrigues V, da Silva JS, Pereira VC, Guerra-Sá R. Epigenetic and parasitological parameters are modulated in EBi3−/− mice infected with *Schistosoma mansoni*. PLoS Neglected Tropical Diseases. 2020;**14**(2):1-24. DOI: 10.1371/journal.pntd.0008080

[15] Costain AH, MacDonald AS, Smits HH. Schistosome egg migration: Mechanisms, pathogenesis and host immune responses. Frontiers in Immunology. 2018;**9**(December):3042. DOI: 10.3389/fimmu.2018.03042

[16] Everts B, Perona-Wright G, Smits HH, Hokke CH, Van Der Ham AJ, Fitzsimmons CM, et al. Omega-1, a glycoprotein secreted by *Schistosoma mansoni* eggs, drives Th2 responses. Journal of Experimental Medicine. 2009;**206**(8):1673-1680. DOI: 10.1084/jem.20082460

[17] Fairfax KC, Amiel E, King IL, Freitas TC, Mohrs M, Pearce EJ. IL-10R blockade during chronic schistosomiasis Mansoni results in the loss of B cells from the liver and the development of severe pulmonary disease. PLoS Pathogens. Jan 2012;**8**(1):e1002490. DOI: 10.1371/journal.ppat.1002490. [Epub Jan 26, 2012]. PMID: 22291593, PMCID: PMC3266936

[18] Zheng B, Zhang J, Chen H, Nie H, Miller H, Gong Q, et al. T lymphocyte-mediated liver immunopathology of schistosomiasis. Frontiers in Immunology. 2020;**11**(February):1-13. DOI: 10.3389/fimmu.2020.00061

[19] Cheeseman K, Weitzman JB. Host-parasite interactions: An intimate epigenetic relationship. Cellular Microbiology. 2015;**17**(8):1121-1132. DOI: 10.1111/cmi.12471

[20] Xiao SH, Sun J, Chen MG. Pharmacological and immunological effects of Praziquantel against *Schistosoma japonicum*: A scoping review of experimental studies. Infectious Diseases of Poverty. 2018;**7**(1):1-15. DOI: 10.1186/s40249-018-0391-x

[21] Frahm S, Anisuzzaman A, Prodjinotho F, Vejzagić N, Verschoor A, da Costa CP. A novel cell-free method to culture *Schistosoma mansoni* from Cercariae to juvenile worm stages for in vitro drug testing. PLoS Neglected Tropical Diseases. 2019;**13**(1):1-22. DOI: 10.1371/journal.pntd.0006590

[22] Langenberg MCC, Hoogerwerf MA, Koopman JPR, Janse JJ, Oosterhoud J K-v, Feijt C, et al. A controlled human *Schistosoma mansoni* infection model to advance novel drugs, vaccines and diagnostics. Nature Medicine. 2020;**26**(3):326-332. DOI: 10.1038/s41591-020-0759-x

[23] Mnkugwe RH, Minzi OS, Kinung'hi SM, Kamuhabwa AA, Aklillu E. Efficacy and safety of praziquantel for treatment of *Schistosoma mansoni* infection among school children in Tanzania. Pathogens. 2019;**9**(1):28. DOI: 10.3390/pathogens9010028. PMID: 31892235, PMCID: PMC7168679

[24] Mwinzi PNM, Kittur N, Ochola E, Cooper PJ, Campbell CH, King CH, et al. Additional evaluation of the point-of-contact circulating cathodic antigen assay for *Schistosoma mansoni* infection. Frontiers in Public Health. 2015;**3**(Mar):1-8. DOI: 10.3389/fpubh.2015.00048

[25] Olliaro P, Delgado-Romero P, Keiser J. The little we know about the pharmacokinetics and pharmacodynamics of praziquantel (Racemate and R-enantiomer). Journal of Antimicrobial Chemotherapy. 2014;**69**(4):863-870. DOI: 10.1093/jac/dkt491

[26] Aruleba RT, Adekiya TA, Oyinloye BE, Masamba P, Mbatha LS, Pretorius A, et al. PZQ therapy: How close are we in the development of effective alternative anti-Schistosomal drugs? Infectious Disorders—Drug Targets. 2019;**19**(4):337-349. DOI: 10.2174/1871526519666181231153139

[27] Abou-El-Naga IF, Amer EI, Boulos LM, El-Faham MH, Abou Seada NM, Younis SS. Biological and proteomic studies of *Schistosoma mansoni* with decreased sensitivity to praziquantel. Comparative Immunology, Microbiology and Infectious Diseases. 2019;**66**(April):101341. DOI: 10.1016/j.cimid.2019.101341

[28] Pica-Mattoccia L, Cioli D. Sex- and stage-related sensitivity of *Schistosoma mansoni* to in vivo and in vitro praziquantel treatment. International Journal for Parasitology. 2004;**34**(4):527-533. DOI: 10.1016/j.ijpara.2003.12.003

[29] Cioli D, Pica-Mattoccia L, Basso A, Guidi A. Schistosomiasis control: Praziquantel forever? Molecular and Biochemical Parasitology. 2014;**195**(1):23-29. DOI: 10.1016/j.molbiopara.2014.06.002

[30] Viana M, Faust CL, Haydon DT, Webster JP, Lamberton PHL. The effects of subcurative praziquantel treatment on life-history traits and trade-offs in drug-resistant *Schistosoma mansoni*. Evolutionary Applications. 2018;**11**(4):488-500. DOI: 10.1111/eva.12558

[31] Tolsma TO, Hansen JC. Post-translational modifications and chromatin dynamics. Essays in Biochemistry. 2019;**63**(1):89-96. DOI: 10.1042/ebc20180067

[32] Fan J, Krautkramer KA, Feldman JL, Denu JM. Metabolic regulation of histone post-translational modifications. ACS Chemical Biology. 2015;**10**(1):95-108. DOI: 10.1021/cb500846u

[33] Fabrizio P, Garvis S, Palladino F. Histone methylation and memory of environmental stress. Cell. 2019;**8**(4):339. DOI: 10.3390/cells8040339

[34] Meas R, Mao P. Histone Ubiquitylation and its roles in transcription and DNA damage response. DNA Repair. 2015;**36**:36-42. DOI: 10.1016/j.dnarep.2015.09.016

[35] Afrin F, Khan I, Hemeg HA. Leishmania-host interactions-an epigenetic paradigm. Frontiers in Immunology. 2019;**10**(March):492. DOI: 10.3389/fimmu.2019.00492

[36] Cosseau C, Wolkenhauer O, Padalino G, Geyer KK, Hoffmann KF, Grunau C. (Epi)genetic inheritance in *Schistosoma mansoni*: A systems approach. Trends in Parasitology. 2017;**33**(4):285-294. DOI: 10.1016/j.pt.2016.12.002

[37] Biswas S, Mallikarjuna Rao C. Epigenetic tools (the writers, the readers and the erasers) and their implications in cancer therapy. European Journal of Pharmacology. 2018;**837**:8-24. DOI: 10.1016/j.ejphar.2018.08.021

[38] Roquis D, Lepesant JMJ, Picard MAL, Freitag M, Parrinello H, Groth M, et al. The epigenome of *Schistosoma mansoni* provides insight about how Cercariae poise transcription until infection. PLoS Neglected Tropical Diseases. 2015;**9**(8):1-22. DOI: 10.1371/journal.pntd.0003853

[39] Roquis D, Taudt A, Geyer KK, Padalino G, Hoffmann KF, Holroyd N, et al. Histone methylation changes are required for life cycle progression in the human parasite *Schistosoma mansoni*. PLoS Pathogens. 2018;**14**(5):1-26. DOI: 10.1371/journal.ppat.1007066

[40] Jeremias WDJ, Araújo FMG, Queiroz FR, Pais FSM, De Mattos ACA, Salim ACDM, et al. Comparative sequence analysis reveals regulation of genes in developing Schistosomula of *Schistosoma mansoni* exposed to host portal serum. PLoS One. 2017;**12**(6):1-19. DOI: 10.1371/journal.pone.0178829

[41] Yun SM, Kim SH, Kim EH. The molecular mechanism of transforming growth factor-β signaling for intestinal fibrosis: A mini-review. Frontiers in Pharmacology. Feb 27 2019;**10**:162. DOI: 10.3389/fphar.2019.00162. PMID: 30873033, PMCID: PMC6400889

[42] Zhang W, Le L, Ahmad G, Molehin AJ, Siddiqui AJ, Torben W, et al. Fifteen years of Sm-P80-based vaccine trials in nonhuman primates: Antibodies from vaccinated baboons confer protection in vivo and in vitro from *Schistosoma mansoni* and identification of putative correlative markers of protection. Frontiers in Immunology. 2020;**11**(June):1-17. DOI: 10.3389/fimmu.2020.01246

[43] Abdulla MH, Ruelas DS, Wolff B, Snedecor J, Lim KC, Xu F, et al. Drug discovery for schistosomiasis: Hit and lead compounds identified in a library of known drugs by medium-throughput phenotypic screening. PLoS Neglected Tropical Diseases. 2009;**3**(7):e478. DOI: 10.1371/journal.pntd.0000478. PMID: 19597541, PMCID: PMC2702839

[44] Aguiar DPD, Moscardini MBM, Morais ER, De Paula RG, Ferreira PM, Afonso A, et al. Curcumin generates oxidative stress and induces apoptosis in adult *Schistosoma mansoni* Worms. PLoS One. 2016;**11**(11):1-25. DOI: 10.1371/journal.pone.0167135

[45] Barban A, Cabral FJ, Luiz A, Bitencourt B, Brigato OM. Inhibition of 19S proteasome deubiquitinating activity in *Schistosoma mansoni* affects viability, oviposition, and structural changes. Parasitology Research. 2020;**119**(7):2159-2176

[46] do Patrocínio B, Andressa FJC, de Paiva TH, Magalhães LG, de Lima Paula LA, Brigato OM, et al. Deubiquitinating enzymes as possible drug targets for schistosomiasis. Acta Tropica. 2021;**217**(February):105856. DOI: 10.1016/j.actatropica.2021.105856. [Epub Feb 9, 2021]. PMID: 33577811

[47] Bibo-Verdugo B, Wang SC, Almaliti J, Ta AP, Jiang Z, Wong DA, et al. The proteasome as a drug target in the metazoan pathogen, *Schistosoma mansoni*. ACS Infectious Diseases. 11 Oct 2019;**5**(10):1802-1812. DOI: 10.1021/acsinfecdis.9b00237. [Epub 12 Aug, 2019]. PMID: 31355632; PMCID: PMC7283364

[48] Crellen T, Allan F, David S, Durrant C, Huckvale T, Holroyd N, et al. Whole genome resequencing of the human parasite *Schistosoma mansoni* reveals population history and effects of selection. Scientific Reports. 2016;**6**(October 2015):1-13. DOI: 10.1038/srep20954

[49] Lucas LA, Cândido ACBB, Santos MFC, Caffrey CR, Bastos JK, Ambrósio SR, et al. Antiparasitic properties of propolis extracts and their compounds. Chemistry and Biodiversity. 2021;**18**(9). DOI: 10.1002/cbdv.202100310

[50] Magalhães LG, Machado CB, Morais ER, Moreira ÉBDC, Soares CS, Da Silva SH, et al. In vitro Schistosomicidal activity of curcumin against *Schistosoma mansoni* adult worms. Parasitology Research. 2009;**104**(5):1197-1201. DOI: 10.1007/s00436-008-1311-y

[51] Qokoyi NK, Masamba P, Kappo AP. Proteins as targets in anti-Schistosomal drug discovery and vaccine development.

Vaccine(Basel). Jul 8 2021;**9**(7):762. DOI: 10.3390/vaccines9070762. PMID: 34358178, PMCID: PMC8310332

[52] Siddiqui. Clinical trials clinical trials. Cancer. 1989;**33**(3):1-2. DOI: 10.1016/j.pt.2016.10.010.Sm-p80-based

[53] Santiago F, De E, De Oliveira SA, Filho GBDO, Moreira DRM, Gomes PAT, et al. Evaluation of the anti-*Schistosoma mansoni* activity of Thiosemicarbazones and Thiazoles. Antimicrobial Agents and Chemotherapy. 2014;**58**(1):352-363. DOI: 10.1128/AAC.01900-13

[54] Augusto R d C, Duval D, Grunau C. Effects of the environment on developmental plasticity and infection success of *Schistosoma* parasites—An epigenetic perspective. Frontiers in Microbiology. 2019;**10**(July):1-9. DOI: 10.3389/fmicb.2019.01475

[55] Carneiro VC, de Abreu da Silva IC, Torres EJL, Caby S, Lancelot J, Vanderstraete M, et al. Epigenetic changes modulate Schistosome egg formation and are a novel target for reducing transmission of schistosomiasis. PLoS Pathogens. 2014;**10**(5):e1004116. DOI: 10.1371/journal.ppat.1004116. PMID: 24809504, PMCID: PMC4014452

[56] Anisuzzaman, Tsuji N. Schistosomiasis and hookworm infection in humans: Disease burden, pathobiology and anthelmintic vaccines. Parasitology International. 2020;**75**(April 2019):102051. DOI: 10.1016/j.parint.2020.102051

[57] Eyayu T, Zeleke AJ, Worku L. Current status and future prospects of protein vaccine candidates against *Schistosoma mansoni* infection. Parasite Epidemiology and Control. 2020;**11**:e00176. DOI: 10.1016/j.parepi.2020.e00176

[58] Ahmad G, Zhang W, Torben W, Haskins C, Diggs S, Noor Z, et al. Prime-boost and recombinant protein vaccination strategies using Sm-P80 protects against *Schistosoma mansoni* infection in the mouse model to levels previously attainable only by the irradiated cercarial vaccine. Parasitology Research. 2009;**105**(6):1767-1777. DOI: 10.1007/s00436-009-1646-z

[59] Rojo JU, Melkus MW, Kottapalli KR, Okiya OE, Sudduth J, Zhang W, et al. Sm-P80-based schistosomiasis vaccine mediated epistatic interactions identified potential immune signatures for vaccine efficacy in mice and baboons. PLoS One. 2017;**12**(2):1-28. DOI: 10.1371/journal.pone.0171677

[60] Wu HW, Park S, Pond-Tor S, Stuart R, Zhou S, Yang H, et al. Whole-proteome differential screening identifies novel vaccine candidates for schistosomiasis japonica. Journal of Infectious Diseases. 2021;**223**(7):1265-1274. DOI: 10.1093/infdis/jiab085

[61] Santini-Oliveira M, Coler RN, Parra J, Veloso V, Jayashankar L, Pinto PM, et al. Schistosomiasis vaccine candidate Sm14/GLA-SE: Phase 1 safety and immunogenicity clinical trial in healthy, male adults. Vaccine. 2016;**34**(4):586-594. DOI: 10.1016/j.vaccine.2015.10.027

[62] Gouveia MJ, Brindley PJ, Gärtner F, Correia JM, Costa D, Vale N. Drug repurposing for schistosomiasis: Combinations of drugs or biomolecules. Pharmaceuticals. 2018;**11**(1):1-34. DOI: 10.3390/ph11010015

[63] Pereira AC, e Silva M LAe, Souza JM, de Laurentiz RS, Rodrigues V, Januário AH, et al. In vitro and in vivo anthelmintic activity of (−)-6,6'-dinitrohinokinin against Schistosomula and juvenile and adult worms of *Schistosoma mansoni*. Acta Tropica. 2015;**149**:195-201. DOI: 10.1016/j.actatropica.2015.06.005

[64] Albuquerque RDDG d, Mahomoodally MF, Lobine D, Suroowan S, Rengasamy KRR. Botanical products in the treatment and control of schistosomiasis: Recent studies and distribution of active plant resources according to affected regions. Biology. 2020;**9**(8):1-26. DOI: 10.3390/biology9080223

[65] El Wahab A, Wegdan M, El-Badry AA, Mahmoud SS, El-Badry YA, El-Badry MA, et al. Ginger (*Zingiber Officinale*)-derived nanoparticles in *Schistosoma mansoni* infected mice: Hepatoprotective and enhancer of etiological treatment. PLoS Neglected Tropical Diseases. 2021;**15**(5):1-17. DOI: 10.1371/journal.pntd.0009423

[66] Lu TX, Rothenberg ME. MicroRNA. Journal of Allergy and Clinical Immunology. 2018;**141**(4):1202-1207. DOI: 10.1016/j.jaci.2017.08.034

[67] Saliminejad K, Khorshid HRK, Fard SS, Ghaffari SH. An overview of MicroRNAs: Biology, functions, therapeutics, and analysis methods. Journal of Cellular Physiology. May 2019;**234**(5):5451-5465. DOI: 10.1002/jcp.27486. [Epub Nov 23, 2018]. PMID: 30471116

[68] Chen Q, Zhang J, Zheng T, Chen H, Nie H, Zheng B, et al. The role of microRNAs in the pathogenesis, grading and treatment of hepatic fibrosis in schistosomiasis. Parasites and Vectors. 2019;**12**(1):1-10. DOI: 10.1186/s13071-019-3866-0